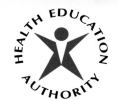

GW00708408

BIRTH
TO FIVE

The Health Education

Authority's complete

guide to the first five

years of being a parent

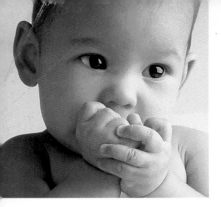

Contents

About this book

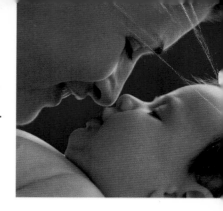

No one needs a book to tell them what's good about being a parent. Parents turn to books when they need information, when they're anxious, when they've got questions or concerns, small or large. This is a book you can turn to.

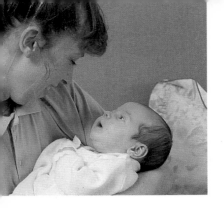

1 The first weeks

'I don't think I'll ever forget those first few days. Feeling so happy, though I don't know why. I couldn't sleep, I was sore, I couldn't move about very well, but I felt happier than I can ever begin to say.'

'There was none of this love at first sight. It was a long time before I came to love him. I can say that now, but at the time I couldn't tell anybody. I thought there was something wrong with me. There was all that work, and feeling rough myself, and because I didn't have this overwhelming feeling for him, none of it made much sense. But oh yes, after three or four months or so of all that, yes, it came right then.'

'I didn't think I'd feel the way I do about her. Sometimes I look at her when she's sleeping, you know, and I have to put my face down next to hers, just to check she's breathing.'

(A FATHER)

There's something very special and exciting about being alone for the first time with your new baby, but it can also be frightening. This is when you begin to realise that you can never go back. You're now responsible for a new human being. The responsibility may seem much too big. You may have a secret wish to run home to your own mother and ask her to take over. Or you may be the kind of person who just knows that you'll get through and that everything will turn out fine in the end.

In these early weeks you'll find there's a great deal to learn, and all of it at the same time. Think of these first few pages as a guide to the basic information you'll need to survive. Today it might seem impossible. In a matter of months you'll look back and wonder how it could have all seemed so hard. Read Chapter 7 for more on how having a baby changes your life.

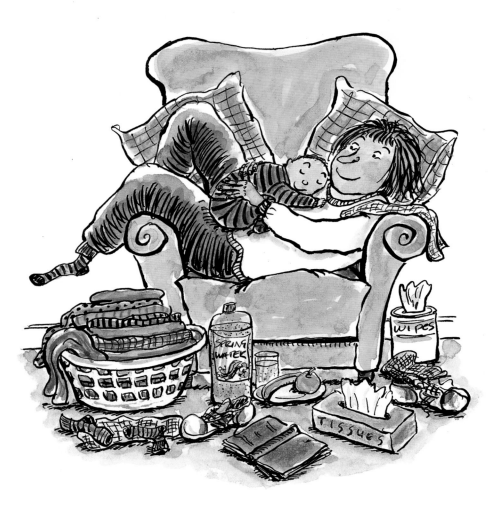

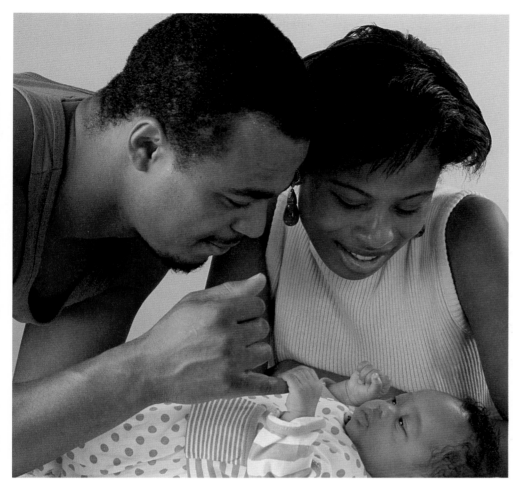

IS IT AN EMERGENCY?

As you get to know your baby you will gain more confidence as a parent and be able to spot when something is wrong more easily. But, in these early days when you are just getting to know your baby, you may not be able to tell what is simply a change from your baby's normal behaviour, or what is a real problem. For instance, is your baby crying because of hunger or colic, or is he or she ill?

If you are worried, never be afraid to ask your midwife, health visitor or GP for help and advice – they are there to help you. See page 81 for how to know when your baby is ill.

COPING WITH THE FIRST FEW WEEKS

- Make your baby your first task and try not to worry about everything else.

- Ask for help from your partner, mother, or friends. Sometimes people with small babies of their own can be the most help because they know what it's like. The health visitor and midwife will also help you to put things into perspective.

- Accept help and suggest to people what they can do: cook a meal and bring it round; do a stack of washing up; do bits of shopping when you run out; take the baby for a walk.

- Sleep whenever your baby allows you to.

- Practice relaxation techniques (see page 117).

- Keep a good supply of nutritious snacks, like fruit, milk, and wholemeal bread, which you can eat without cooking.

- See friends when *you* want to and, if you're tired, tell your friends and suggest that they leave and come back later.

- Remember, this period is hard but it lasts for a relatively short time and it does get better.

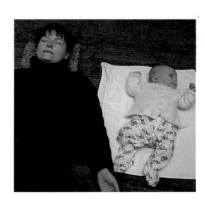

IS IT THE BLUES OR POSTNATAL DEPRESSION?

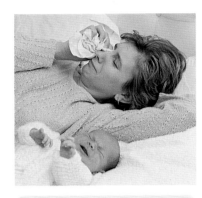

Two organisations that offer help are the Association for Postnatal Illness and the Meet-a-Mum Association (MAMA): their addresses are on page 133. Both organisations will put you in touch with other mothers who've been depressed themselves and know what it's like. Remember that what's called postnatal depression can happen a long time after the birth of a baby.

'Friends kept telling me how well I was coping and I felt really proud. I wanted to be a coping person but underneath I felt I wasn't. And I couldn't admit it either. When I finally talked about it to friends, I found out that a lot of them felt the same way.'

THE BABY BLUES

During the first week after childbirth, most women get what is often called the 'baby blues'. Symptoms can include feeling emotional and irrational, bursting into tears for no apparent reason, feeling irritable or touchy or feeling depressed or anxious. All these symptoms are normal and usually only last for a few days. They are probably due to the sudden hormone and chemical changes which take place in your body after childbirth.

PUERPERAL PSYCHOSIS

One or two mothers in 1000 will also develop an obvious severe psychiatric illness after the birth of their baby, which requires hospital treatment. Usually a complete recovery is made, although this may take a few weeks or months.

POSTNATAL DEPRESSION

This lies between the baby blues and puerperal psychosis, and is an extremely distressing condition with many symptoms. Postnatal depression is thought to affect at least one in ten women, but many women suffer in silence or the condition may go unnoticed by health professionals.

Postnatal depression usually occurs two to eight weeks after delivery. In some cases the baby blues do not go away or the depression can appear up to six months or even a year after the birth of the baby. Some symptoms such as tiredness, irritability or poor appetite are normal if you have just had a baby, but usually these are mild and do not stop you leading a normal life. With postnatal depression you may feel increasingly depressed and despondent and looking after yourself or the baby may become too much. Some other signs of postnatal depression are:

● anxiety

● panic attacks

● sleeplessness

● aches and pains or feeling unwell

● memory loss or unable to concentrate

● can't stop crying

● feelings of hopelessness

● loss of interest in the baby

If you think that you are suffering from postnatal depression don't struggle on alone. It is not a sign that you are a 'bad mother' or are unable to cope. Postnatal depression is an illness just as any other illness. Ask for help just as you would if you had the flu or had broken your leg. Talk to someone you can trust such as your partner or a friend or ask your health visitor to call. It is also important to see your GP – if you don't feel up to making an appointment, ask someone to do this for you, or arrange for him to call. You may also find it helpful to contact the Association for Postnatal Illness, Meet-A-Mum Association (MAMA) or the National Childbirth Trust (see page 133) (see also feeling depressed, on page 118).

BREASTFEEDING

WHY BREASTFEED?

There is no doubt that breastfeeding is best for the health of your baby. As the box on this page shows, it gives him or her many benefits that bottle feeding is unable to provide. If your baby is born prematurely then it's even more beneficial. And there are advantages for you too (see box on page 8). Even if you only breastfeed for a few weeks, your baby will benefit, although the longer you can breastfeed for, the greater the benefits. So, if you are undecided about breastfeeding, why not give it a try? Although you may not find it easy to start with, most difficulties can be overcome with patience and perseverance and, once breastfeeding is established, most mums find they really enjoy it. And you may, of course, find you have no problems at all.

SUCCESSFUL BREASTFEEDING

Understanding how your breasts produce milk and how to deal with any problems that may arise can help you to breastfeed successfully. The next few pages give you lots of information about this.

Your milk supply

Your breasts produce milk in response to your baby feeding at your breast. The more your baby feeds, the more milk you produce provided that your baby is correctly positioned (see **Finding the right position – for your baby** on page 9). So, if you let your baby feed whenever he or she wants to feed, you're likely to produce the amount of milk your baby needs. This is known as demand feeding and at first you may find that your baby will want to feed at two hourly intervals.

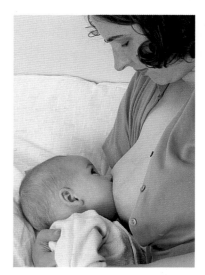

'There's nothing in the world more satisfying than to sit in a darkened silent room, in the middle of the night with a warm baby in your arms, sucking contentedly.'

'I suppose I'd thought that I'd just put her to my breast and that would be it. I hadn't thought of it as something I might have to learn about and practice. So it came as a bit of a shock that the first few weeks were really quite tough. But I was determined I was going to do it, and yes, it's lovely now.'

'I was quite tense at first. I worried whether I was doing it right, and whether I was giving her enough, and I was feeling a bit weepy anyway. You need to find somebody to help and give you confidence. Maybe I was lucky, but my midwife was fantastic. And once I'd got her help, I just relaxed about the whole thing.'

BEST FOR BABY

- *Breast milk is the only food **naturally** designed for your baby and contains all the nutrients your baby needs in the right proportions.*
- *Breast milk contains antibodies and other protective factors which are transferred from you to your baby to help him or her fight against infections. It also helps to build up long-term resistance to infections. Babies who are breastfed are less likely to have gastroenteritis, ear infections, coughs or colds.*
- *Breast milk is easily digested and absorbed and it is less likely to cause stomach upsets or diarrhoea. It will also help to avoid constipation in your baby.*
- *Breastfed babies are less likely to develop allergies such as eczema and asthma.*
- *Breast milk contains factors and other substances which help your baby's growth and development. Formula milks manufactured from cow's milk and used for bottle feeding don't contain any of these living factors, which you alone can provide for your baby.*
- *Breastfeeding may help to prevent **juvenile diabetes** in children who are genetically susceptible to this.*
- *Some studies have found that children who are breastfed have better dental health and better eyesight.*
- *Very tiny premature babies who are given breast milk are more likely to do well.*
- *Breastfed babies may be easier to wean because they are already having traces of what you eat and drink through your breast milk.*

BEST FOR YOU

- *The extra fat laid down by your body during pregnancy is used up when breast milk is made. This can help you get your shape back sooner. (But it is important not to diet when breastfeeding.)*

- *Breastfeeding helps your womb to contract and return to its usual size more quickly.*

- *Breastfeeding for three months or more may reduce the risk of developing breast or ovarian cancer later.*

- *Breastfeeding is practical. There's no cost of preparation and the milk is always available at the right temperature – even in the middle of the night.*

HINTS FOR BREASTFEEDING

- *Eat when you feel hungry, and choose healthy snacks.*

- *Ensure you drink plenty especially in hot weather.*

- *Eat a wide variety of foods; see page 10.*

- *Try not to restrict your diet unless you think a food is upsetting your baby and then talk to your health visitor or doctor before cutting out foods.*

- *Keep your intake of alcohol low – it can unsettle your baby. Avoid drinking shortly before a baby's feed.*

- *Avoid drinking too much strong tea or coffee.*

Don't be tempted to give your baby a bottle at this stage, as this can reduce the time your baby spends sucking at your breast and therefore reduce the milk supply. Your baby may also get confused between sucking from a bottle teat and sucking from your nipple.

Different kinds of breast milk

For the first few days after birth your breasts produce a special food called 'colostrum', which looks like rich creamy milk and is sometimes quite yellow in colour. This contains all the food your baby needs, as well as antibodies which pass your own resistance to certain infections on to your baby.

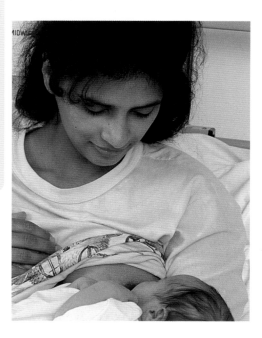

After about three days your breasts will begin to produce milk, which will be quite thin compared with colostrum. Two different kinds of milk are now produced each time you feed your baby. The **fore milk**, which your baby takes first, is thirst quenching and means your baby gets a drink at the start of every feed. This is followed by the richer **hind milk**, which is the food part of the feed and contains the calories your baby needs.

The 'let-down' reflex

Your baby's sucking causes the 'let-down' of your milk. It makes your milk flow down and gather behind your nipple ready for feeding. Sometimes this happens even before your baby starts to feed, maybe when you hear your baby cry. In the early weeks, milk may start to leak from your breasts.

How your baby feeds

Unlike the teat or a bottle, there's no milk in the nipple itself. The breasts are never empty, but the milk has to be let down so that it can gather behind the nipple and areola (the dark area around the nipple). A baby who only sucks on the nipple doesn't get much milk (and may hurt your nipples). To make the milk flow out, your baby has to be in the right position at your breast

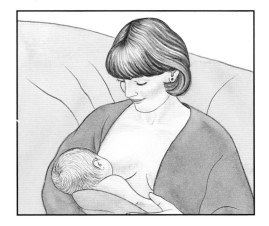

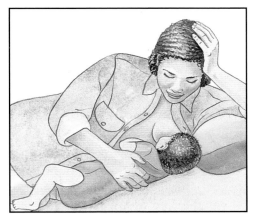

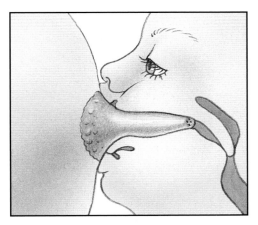

(see above). Make sure your baby's mouth is wide open and covers most of the brown area around your nipple. Your baby's tongue will press the milk out from the milk glands underneath the nipple. When your baby is correctly positioned and the milk begins to flow, you will usually see quick sucks change to deep swallows. Breastfed babies usually pause while they wait for more milk to be 'delivered' rather than sucking non-stop. Look at the pictures on this page to give you a clearer idea.

FINDING THE RIGHT POSITION

For you

Make yourself comfortable. You'll need to hold your baby close to your breast without strain and for some time too, so do make sure that your back is well supported all the way down. Try different chairs and different ways of sitting, and perhaps a footstool to raise your legs. Try lying down on your side with your baby up against you. Find what's best for you.

Later, you won't have to think about what position you're in. You'll be able to feed almost however and wherever you want to.

For your baby

Take your baby up to your breast rather than trying to bring your breast to your baby. Try using a pillow to raise your baby higher.

Hold your baby close and turned towards you with the head and shoulders directly opposite your breast and the nose opposite your nipple. Your baby's back should be in a straight line. Support your baby with a hand across the shoulders, not behind the head. Next, move your baby's lips gently against your nipple to get the baby to open his or her mouth. When the mouth is opened wide, draw the baby to your breast quickly. The baby's bottom lip should reach your breast first.

It's important for your baby to take in your nipple and as much of the brown skin surrounding the nipple as possible. If your baby is correctly positioned, there will be more of your areola showing above the top lip than below the bottom lip, but this is not always easy to see.

Your baby's chin should now be against your breast with the lower lip turned out. It's the baby's lower jaw which does the work of feeding.

If it doesn't feel right, or if it hurts, slide one of your fingers into

SOME SUGGESTED
SNACK FOODS

- *Sandwiches or pitta bread filled with salad vegetables, grated cheese, mashed salmon or sardines*

- *Yoghurts and fromage frais*

- *Hummus and bread or vegetable sticks.*

- *Ready to eat apricots, figs, or prunes.*

- *Vegetable and bean soups.*

- *Fortified unsweetened breakfast cereals with milk.*

- *Milky drinks or unsweetened fruit juices.*

- *Fresh fruit.*

- *Baked beans on toast or baked potato.*

HUNGER OR THIRST?

Breast milk is drink and food in one. If the weather is hot, your baby may want to feed more often. There's no need to give your baby drinks of water even in a very hot climate.

your baby's mouth to gently break the suction and try again. Keep trying until it feels right and you can see your baby taking deep swallows.

YOUR DIET WHEN BREASTFEEDING

Eating well and resting when you can are important in making breast milk. Although your body uses up fat stored during pregnancy, you need extra calories, vitamins, and minerals to keep up with the demands of your growing baby.

It is not wise to restrict your diet whilst breastfeeding even if you are very keen to get back into your normal clothes. Your body is working hard to make milk and needs easily available sources of energy (that is, your diet) to do so. Trying to diet will only make you feel more tired. Eating larger quantities at mealtimes and regular snacks will help meet the additional demands of breastfeeding. Rather than snacking on biscuits and cakes, try to eat foods that are more nutritious such as a sandwich or fruit (see box **Some suggested snack foods**).

Limiting your diet
There should be no need to avoid eating any foods, but if you, your baby's father or any previous children have a history of hayfever, asthma, eczema or other allergies, avoid eating peanuts and foods containing peanut products (e.g. peanut butter, **unrefined** groundnut oils and some snacks). Read food labels carefully and if you are still in doubt about the contents, you should avoid these products.

Some breastfed babies seem to react to foods that their mother has eaten and may cry more as a result. Foods commonly blamed for this

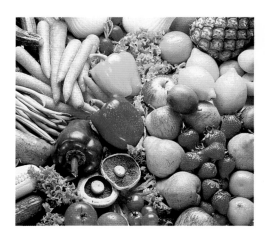

include onions, garlic, citrus fruits and grapes. If you think it might help to cut out these foods, check with your health visitor first. It is important to seek advice before omitting food from your diet, as it is possible to become deficient in certain vitamins and minerals if you don't know which foods to replace them with.

Drinks containing caffeine can unsettle your baby so keep your intake of tea and coffee low. Small amounts of alcohol pass into breastmilk, making it smell different to your baby, and may affect his or her feeding, sleeping, or digestion. So it is best to keep well below the daily limits of two to three units for women, and avoid drinking before you feed your baby.

Milk and dairy products are sometimes said to make breastfed babies upset, but don't cut these out of your diet without medical advice, as they provide the calcium you and your baby need.

HOW OFTEN, HOW LONG?

Some babies settle into a pattern of feeding quite quickly. Others take longer. In the early weeks, you may find that your baby's feeds are sometimes long, sometimes short, sometimes close together, and sometimes further apart. Try to follow what your baby tells you. Feed when your baby asks to be fed, and for as long as your baby wants.

Once you've put your baby to your breast, let the feed go on until your baby wants to stop. Then, either straight away or after a pause, offer the other breast to see if your baby wants more. If you swap from one breast to the other before your baby is ready, you may only be giving your baby the thinner fore milk from each breast. The hind milk which comes later is richer and contains calories that your baby needs (see page 8).

Allow your baby to decide when he or she has had enough. Both breasts might not always be wanted at each feed. Your baby will show that he or she has finished by either letting go of your breast or falling asleep. Start each feed on alternate breasts so that your breasts are stimulated to make milk equally – this should prevent engorgement (see page 12). You could remind yourself which breast was used last by tying a ribbon or pinning a safety pin to the bra strap on the side you last used. Some mothers can tell simply by feeling to see which breast is more full.

If you feed as often and for as long as your baby wants, you'll produce plenty of milk and give your baby what he or she needs. While your baby is very young, this may mean quite lengthy feeds. But if you've got your baby in the right position at your breast, you shouldn't become sore.

At first it may seem that you're doing nothing but feeding. Remember that this stage will not last very long. In time you'll find that your milk supply increases and so will the speed with which your baby feeds. Babies have growth spurts at approximately ten days, six weeks and three months. Your baby may feed more frequently at these times until your milk supply increases to meet the bigger demand.

HOW MUCH IS ENOUGH?

Since it's impossible to see how much milk your baby is taking from your breast, you may wonder whether your baby is getting enough. If you feed as frequently and for as long as your baby wants, you'll find that your baby will stop feeding when he or she is full-up. You can be sure your baby is getting enough milk if he or she:

● has plenty of wet nappies each day and is having nothing but breast milk;

● is growing and generally gaining weight. It is overall weight gain that is important – some babies gain weight steadily, other perfectly healthy babies gain little or no weight one week, then feed more often and make up for it over the next week or two (see pages 37-38);

● is awake and alert for some of the time.

If you notice that your baby isn't growing in length or generally gaining weight, and is very sleepy or lethargic with no alert times, then he or she may not be getting enough milk. Persistent green stools may also be an indication that your baby is getting too much fore milk and not enough of the high calorie hind milk. Always make sure that your baby empties one breast completely before offering the other breast. If you are concerned, talk to your midwife or health visitor. Night feeds are important. A small baby can receive as much milk at night as during the day and night feeds encourage the body to make more of the hormone that produces breast milk. When your baby is small it's important for night feeds to continue.

If your baby seems unusually sleepy and is slow to start feeding, he or she may be ill, so contact your GP.

TWINS

Twins can be breastfed successfully. If you have twins it may help to start feeding each of your twins separately until feeding is well established. Then it may be more convenient to try and encourage them to feed at the same time. Your milk supply will increase to meet this extra demand, but you may need help putting your babies to the breast at the start.

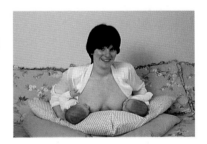

As well as your midwife or health visitor, breastfeeding counsellors from organisations such as La Leche League, *the* National Childbirth Trust, *and the* Association for Breastfeeding Mothers *can provide help and support (see page 133).*

'My nipples hurt when she feeds. What can I do?'
During the first week or two, some breastfeeding mothers feel some discomfort as their baby starts sucking at the beginning of a feed. As soon as the milk begins to flow this discomfort stops. If feeding hurts, your baby's position is probably wrong (see page 9) but if you can't get the position right yourself, ask for help.

'I've been feeding my baby for two weeks now, but my nipple is cracked and painful. Should I give up?'
If your baby is in the right position at your breast, feeding shouldn't hurt.

● Check that your baby is 'fixing' properly. Ask for help if you need it. Once your baby is positioned correctly cracks should heal rapidly.

● Keep your nipples clean and dry, but avoid soap, which dries the skin too much.

● Change breast pads frequently. Avoid pads with plastic backing.

● Wear a cotton bra and let the air get to your nipples as much as possible.

● Try sleeping topless, with a towel under you if you're leaking milk.

● A few drops of milk rubbed into the nipple at the end of a feed may help.

● Thrush in your baby's mouth can sometimes cause sore nipples. Thrush is an infection that results in small white patches in the baby's mouth, which don't wipe away. If you think your baby has

thrush, both you and your baby will need medical treatment, so see your GP.

● If your nipples remain sore, ask a health visitor or breastfeeding counsellor for advice (see box on opposite page).

'He stops and starts and cries and just doesn't seem to settle down.'
If your baby is restless at your breast and doesn't seem satisfied by feeds, he or she may be sucking on the nipple alone and not getting enough milk. Check your baby is in the right position and fixed properly to your breast. Ask for help if you need to. Colic may also be a problem (see page 23).

'My breasts are very swollen and hard and painful. What's wrong?'
Your breasts are 'engorged' which means that they are full of either blood or milk. The first type of engorgement can happen during the first few days before you start to produce milk. It is caused by the blood supply to your breasts increasing as your breasts get ready to make milk. Ask your midwife what to do. She might suggest relieving the discomfort by taking paracetamol.

The second type of engorgement is caused by milk and can happen at any time from about the third day after the birth of your baby, when you start to produce milk. This type of engorgement is common in the first few weeks or if your baby has gone a long time between feeds. The answer is to feed your baby. If feeding is difficult for some reason, ask for help. To ease the swelling, try a hot bath or bathe your breasts with some warm water. Smooth out some milk with your fingers, stroking gently downwards towards the nipple. Or try holding a face cloth wrung out in very cold water against your breast. Check your bra's not too tight.

'I have a hard, painful lump in my breast. What is it?'

It's probably a blocked milk duct. Milk builds up because the ducts aren't being emptied properly. Check that your bra isn't too tight and that nothing is pressing into your breast as you feed (your bra or arm, for example).

A good feed on the blocked breast will help. As you feed, smooth the milk away from the blockage towards the nipple. If this doesn't work, ask for help. If left untreated, blocked ducts can lead to mastitis (see below).

'There is a red, hot, painful patch on my breast and I feel quite unwell. Why?'

You may have mastitis. Don't stop feeding as you need to keep your milk moving. Try different positions to empty different parts of your breast. Try the suggestions for relieving engorged breasts and blocked ducts, get lots of rest, and try not to wear a bra, especially at night. A health visitor or breastfeeding counsellor can offer information, help and support. You may also need antibiotics to clear the infection. Your doctor can prescribe one that is safe to take while breastfeeding.

'My milk looks thin and is a different colour to bottle milk.'

There is a great variation in the colour and consistency of breastmilk. Unlike bottled milk, the cream is at the bottom and not the top! The first part of the milk, the fore milk, is thirst - quenching and may look watery and bluish. The second part, the hind milk, is thicker and can vary from creamy white to yellowish. Your baby doesn't mind the colour.

MAKING BREASTFEEDING WORK FOR YOU

Some mothers are happy to feed anywhere and in front of anyone. That's fine. Other mothers like being able to breastfeed, but are uncomfortable with the idea of exposing themselves in public. However, it is possible to breastfeed

HELP WITH BREASTFEEDING

You can get help and advice from:

- *your community midwife, health visitor or GP;*

- *a breastfeeding counsellor or support group. Contact your local branch of the National Childbirth Trust, La Leche League or the Association of Breastfeeding Mothers (see page 133). These organisations can provide you with help and support from other mothers with experience of breastfeeding.*

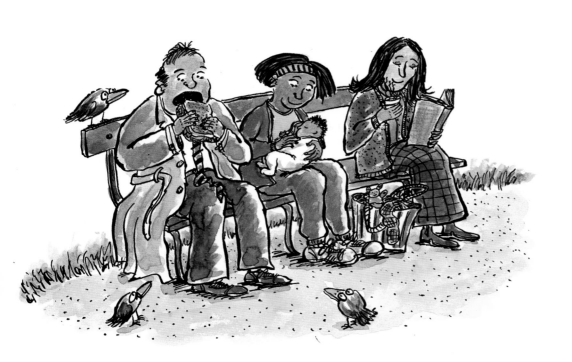

If you are able to breastfeed for at least four months your baby will have the best start in life. Try just to give breastmilk as giving formula or water can decrease the benefit.

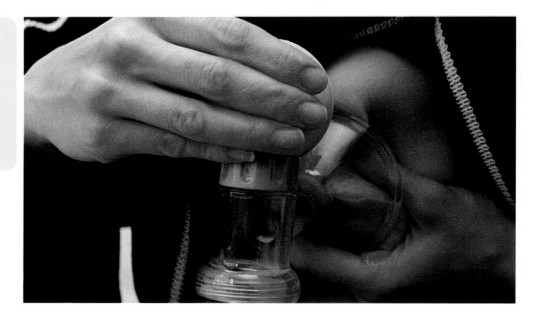

discreetly. You can choose clothes that make it easy, such as a loose top or T-shirt that you can pull upwards. Practising in front of a mirror before you go out might help you to feel more confident.

If you simply find the idea of breastfeeding in front of others awkward and embarrassing, you might prefer to live a very private life for the first few months with your baby. That's fine too. Don't feel under pressure to socialise if you don't want to. When you do go out, ask if there is another room where you can feed your baby. Many shops and public places now provide mothers' rooms. Do what feels best for you.

EXPRESSING MILK

If you want to express milk in the first few weeks (perhaps because your baby is in Special Care), ask your midwife about it. Hospitals often keep machines for people who need to express milk and you can be shown how to use it. Alternatively, the Association of Breastfeeding Mothers, La Leche League and the National Childbirth Trust all have breast pumps for hire (see page 133).

Unless there's a special reason for expressing milk, it's usually easier not to try it until you've got breastfeeding well established. After six weeks or so you may want to express milk for someone else to give to your baby.

If you've plenty of milk you'll probably find expressing quite easy, particularly if you do it in the morning. However, some mothers do find it quite difficult. Your midwife or health visitor will show you how to express milk either using an electric or hand pump or by hand.

You must express your milk into a sterilised bottle, which you can then cap and keep in the fridge. Don't keep it for longer than 24 hours. You can also freeze breast milk if you want to keep it for a few weeks, but make sure you freeze it as soon as possible after expressing it, and certainly within a couple of hours (there are specially designed breast milk freezer bags). When you want to use it, put it in the fridge until completely defrosted but then treat it as you would bottled milk (see pages 16-18).

If the father wants to become involved in feeding, he can give your expressed milk to the baby.

COMBINING BREAST AND BOTTLE

In the early weeks

If you want to breastfeed it's best to completely avoid giving bottles to your baby in the early weeks. This is especially true if you don't think you're producing enough milk – your baby needs to breastfeed frequently to make sure there is enough milk. However, if you are concerned that you're not producing enough milk for your baby, contact your health visitor or lay breastfeeding counsellor for help **before** you decide to give a bottle.

If you do eventually decide to give the occasional bottle, but then would like to go back to full breastfeeding, you can, but you will have to breastfeed your baby often and for longer to increase your milk supply. Feeds will space out again once your milk supply has increased. Of course, weaning your baby off the breast might be the right answer for you, especially if breastfeeding is making you unhappy.

Once breastfeeding is well established

You've more flexibility for combining breast and bottle at this later stage. You can introduce a regular bottle feed of formula milk if, for example, you're returning to work or simply want someone else involved in feeding. If you offer the bottle feed at the same time each day, your own supply will adjust quite quickly and you should be able to keep on breastfeeding at the other feeds. Mothers returning to work, for example, often breastfeed in the morning and evening and their babies have a cup or bottle of formula during the day (see pages 16–18).

CHANGING FROM BREAST TO BOTTLE

If you're having difficulty breastfeeding and decide to change to bottle feeding, you're unlikely to experience difficulty getting your baby to take a bottle and you'll probably both feel more relaxed when feeding settles down. If you have been breastfeeding exclusively, but now need to get your baby to take a bottle, perhaps because you're returning to work or for some other reason, then you may find it difficult at first.

It might be easier to change over to infant formula using a cup or egg cup. There is no reason why you *have* to use a bottle. Don't stop breastfeeding suddenly as this can cause your breasts to become hard, swollen and uncomfortable). Give yourself time for the changeover and cut out one feed at a time, starting well before your return to work. It's probably best not to give the first bottle feed at times when your baby is tired and it may help if someone other than you gives the first feeds. Your baby is not then near your breast, smelling and expecting breast milk. Don't panic if you experience difficulties at first. Your baby will get used to the new arrangements in time. If you are concerned that your baby is not getting enough milk, see **How much is enough?** on page 11.

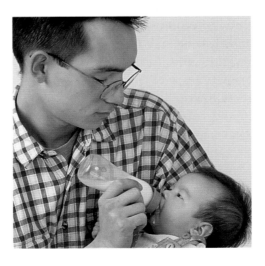

BOTTLE FEEDING

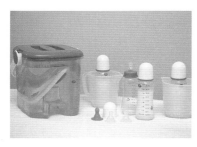

Get well organised for bottle feeding so that you can enjoy it. In time, you'll find your own routine for preparing feeds and sterilising.

WHAT YOU'LL NEED

- **At least six bottles and teats –** there are different kinds of bottles and teats. Ask your midwife, health visitor, or other mothers if you want advice on what to buy. You may be offered secondhand bottles. Make sure they're not scratched – if they are, you won't be able to sterilise them properly. Always buy new teats.

- **A supply of baby milk** – there are lots of different brands of baby milk (also called 'infant formula') marketed in different ways. Some milks contain fats called long chain polyunsaturates like breast milk, some are said to be suitable for hungrier bottle-fed babies, or are labelled 'first milk' or 'second milk'. Looking at this choice you may well be confused what milk to use. However, all baby milks marketed in the UK have to comply with rigorous legislation, and have to contain certain levels of protein, carbohydrate, fats, vitamins and minerals, although different types of fats and carbohydrates may be used. Ideally, discuss the different brands with your midwife or health visitor and then make your own choice, based on this information. Sometimes a hospital may also recommend a certain brand of milk if your baby was premature and you can't manage to breastfeed.

  If there is a strong history of allergies in your family, such as eczema, asthma or food allergies (known as 'atopic disease'), and you think you won't manage to breastfeed, seek advice as early as possible from your GP or health visitor. You may be referred to a paediatrician or a doctor who has a special interest in allergies. If your baby has an allergic reaction to milk formula it may be necessary to use non-dairy (soya-based) milks. But don't change to non-dairy baby milks without talking to your doctor or health visitor first because they can also trigger allergies. Unmodified goat's milk or sheep's milk are not nutritionally suitable for babies under one year of age.

  Milk is usually sold cheaply in clinics but can be cheaper still in large supermarkets, so it's worth comparing prices. If you are on benefits see page 129 to check whether you can claim free or low price milk for your baby.

- **Sterilising equipment** (see page 17).

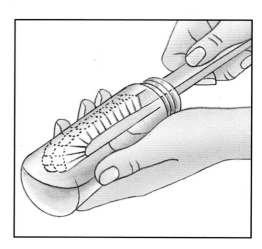

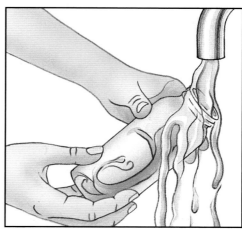

MAKING UP FEEDS

- *Always wash your hands with soap and water before you start.*

- *To make up milk, always put the water in first and then follow exactly the instructions on the tin or packet. Don't add extra powder or anything else, like baby rice, as it will become too strong and your baby may not be able to digest it properly. In some cases this could make him or her ill.*

- *You can make up a day's feeds in advance and store the capped bottles in the fridge. This saves time, and means you don't have to make your baby wait while you make up a feed - although you will need six or seven bottles and teats. Don't keep the made-up milk for longer than 24 hours and shake the bottle well before you use it.*

- *If your baby doesn't finish a bottle, don't keep the extra. Throw it away.*

WASHING AND STERILISING

Your bottles and teats must be washed and sterilised until your baby is at least six months old to protect against infection.

Washing
Wash your baby's bottles and teats thoroughly using washing-up liquid. Usually, salt is no longer recommended for cleaning teats, but if you are advised to use salt, use as little as possible and make sure you rinse it off thoroughly. Make sure you get rid of every trace of milk, squirting water through the teats and using a bottle brush for the bottles. Rinse in clean water.

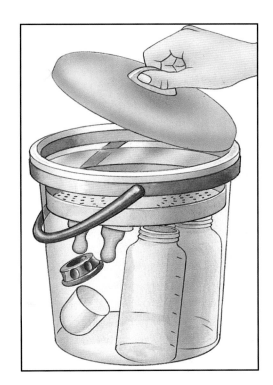

Sterilising
There are a number of different ways of sterilising.

Chemical sterilising You can buy a complete sterilising unit in the shops or use a plastic bucket with a lid.

- To make up the solution, follow the instructions that come with the sterilising tablets or liquid.

- Immerse your baby's washed bottles, lids and teats in sterilising solution. Leave them in the solution for the time given in the instructions. If you're using a bucket, keep everything under the water by putting a plate on top. Make sure there aren't any air bubbles inside the bottles and don't add any other unsterilised things to the container later or you will have to start all over again.

- When you take the bottles and teats out to make up your baby's feeds, wash your own hands first. Don't rinse the bottles and teats with tap water because you'll make them unsterile again. If you want to rinse off the sterilising solution, use boiled, cooled water.

Sterilising by boiling
- Put washed equipment into a large pan with a lid. Make sure no air is trapped in the bottles.

- Boil for at least ten minutes (teats need just three). Leave everything in the covered pan until needed.

- Keep the pan out of the reach of older children.

- Keep your pan only for sterilising this equipment.

- Teats that are boiled regularly get sticky and need replacing regularly.

Steam sterilisers There are steam sterilisers specially designed for bottles which are both quick and efficient.

Microwave steam units These steam units are designed specifically for sterilising bottles in a microwave oven. If you intend to sterilise bottles in a microwave oven you must use one of these units, otherwise 'cold spots' may occur and could leave part of the bottle unsterilised.

FEEDING

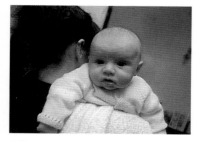

BOTTLE FEEDING HELP
AND ADVICE

*If you want help or advice
on bottle feeding, talk to
your midwife or health
visitor, or to other mothers
with experience of bottle
feeding.*

*'I wouldn't have missed it.
When he was small, those
feeds brought us close.
It was how we got to
know each other.'*

(A FATHER)

*'Early on, if the feeds weren't
going well, I'd think, well,
perhaps I'd better try a different
kind of milk, or a different
bottle, or a different teat, or
whatever. But it's the same as
doing anything the first time.
It's a while before you know
what you're doing, and then
you settle down and
start to enjoy it.'*

- You can warm your baby's bottle before a feed by standing it in some hot water. Test the temperature of the milk by squirting some on to your wrist. Some babies don't mind cold milk, others like it warmed. Don't give a baby milk that has been kept warm for more than an hour before a feed – germs breed in the warmth. It's dangerous to use a microwave oven to warm a bottle of milk. The milk continues to heat for a time after you take it out of the microwave, although the outside of the bottle may feel cold.

- Get yourself comfortable so that you can cuddle your baby close as you feed. Give your baby time, and let him or her take as much milk as he or she wants. Some babies take some milk and drop off to sleep, then wake up for more. Be patient. At the end of a feed throw away any leftover milk.

- As you feed, keep the bottle tilted so that the teat is always full of milk, otherwise your baby will be taking in air.

- If the teat flattens while you're feeding, pull gently on the bottle to release the vacuum. If the teat blocks, start again with another sterile teat.

- Teats come in all sorts of shapes and with different hole sizes. You may need to experiment to find the right teat and hole size for your baby. If the hole's too small, your baby will suck and suck without getting enough milk. If it's too big, your baby will get too much too quickly and probably spit and splutter or bring the feed back. A small teat hole can be made larger with a red-hot needle if the teat is made of latex. If it is made of silicone you shouldn't try to enlarge the hole – it is more likely to tear, and bits could break off into your baby's mouth.

- **Never prop up a bottle and leave your baby to feed alone –** he or she may choke.

- Don't add solids to bottle feeds. Your baby can't digest them and may choke.

WIND – AND WHAT MAY COME WITH IT

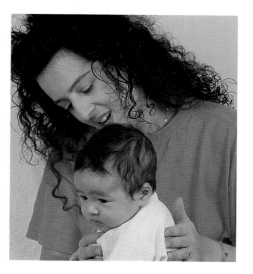

If your baby swallows a lot of air while feeding and is then put down to sleep, the trapped wind may cause discomfort and your baby may cry. After a feed, it may help to hold your baby upright against your shoulder or propped forward on your lap. Then gently rub your baby's back so that any trapped air can find its way up and out quite easily. Some babies are never troubled by wind, others seem to suffer discomfort after every feed. For information about colic, see pages 23–24.

Some babies sick up more milk than others during or just after a feed. (This is called 'possetting', 'regurgitation' or 'gastric reflux'.) It's not unusual for a baby to sick up quite a lot, but many mothers get upset or worried about this. If your baby is gaining weight there is usually nothing to worry about. But if this happens often or if your baby is frequently or violently sick, appears to be in pain, or you're worried for any other reason, see your health visitor or GP.
Cover your baby with a thick bib when feeding and have a cloth or paper towels handy to mop up any mess. (If you sprinkle a damp cloth with bicarbonate of soda this will remove the worst of the smell.) Check too that the hole in your baby's teat is not too big. Sitting your baby upright in a baby chair after a feed can help, and the problem usually stops by the age of six months when your baby is taking more solids and drinking less milk. If your baby brings back a lot of milk, remember he or she is likely to be hungry again quite quickly. If the reflux is severe, your GP or health visitor may recommend a powder to thicken the milk.

SLEEPING

Some babies sleep much more than others. Some sleep in long patches, some in short. Some soon sleep right through the night, some don't for a long time. Your baby will have his or her own pattern of waking and sleeping, and it's unlikely to be the same as other babies you know. Also, the pattern will change over time.

One thing is certain. In the early weeks your baby's sleeping pattern is very unlikely to fit in with your need for sleep. Try to follow your baby's needs. You'll gradually get to know when sleep is needed. Don't catch up on housework while your baby sleeps. Snatch sleep and rest whenever you can.

A baby who wants to sleep isn't likely to be disturbed by household noise. So there's no need to keep the house silent while your baby sleeps. In fact, it will help you if your child gets used to sleeping through a certain amount of noise.

Most parents want their children to learn to sleep for the longest period at night – when they are sleeping – and it helps if you encourage night-time sleeping right from the start by teaching your baby that the night-time is different from the daytime. During night feeds:

- keep the lights down low;

- keep your voice low and don't talk much;

- put your baby down as soon as you have fed and changed him or her;

- don't change your baby if a change is not needed.

If your baby always falls asleep in your arms, at your breast, in your partner's arms, or with someone by the cot, he or she might not easily take to settling alone. This might not matter to you and may be unavoidable in the early weeks, particularly with a breastfed baby. But, if you want your baby to get used to going off to sleep alone, it's wise to start right from the beginning, by putting the baby down before he or she falls asleep whenever this is possible. However, you may need to wait until the baby is alert for longer or more frequent periods. Remember though, the longer you leave it, the more difficult it will become.

Once you've established a pattern you may want to try and shift things around a bit. For example, you may wake your baby for a feed just before you go to bed in the hope that you'll get a good long stretch of sleep

'It wasn't that she wouldn't sleep when she needed to. She just didn't need it. Or at least, she needed a whole lot less than we did. It's not getting your baby to sleep that's the problem; it's getting enough sleep yourself.'

'I would just get one of them off to sleep when the other one woke for a feed. I was desperately tired but gradually they got into a pattern and at last I could get some sleep myself.'

Don't leave your baby alone with a bottle as a way of getting him or her off to sleep. There's a danger of choking.

Disturbed nights can be very hard to bear. If you're bottle feeding, encourage your partner to share the feeds. Many fathers find this a valuable time for getting to know their babies. If you're breastfeeding, your partner may be happy to take over the early morning changing and dressing so that you can go back to sleep, or once breastfeeding is established he could occasionally give a bottle of expressed breast milk. If you're on your own, you could ask a friend or relative to stay for a few days so that you can sleep.

If your baby seems at all unwell, seek medical advice early and quickly. Do remember that cot death is rare. Don't let worrying about cot death spoil the first precious months you have with your baby.

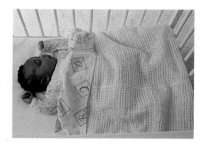

before he or she wakes again.

See pages 54–56 for more information about sleeping problems in older babies and children. Serene (formerly known as CRY-SIS), the organisation for parents of crying babies, can also offer help with sleeping problems (address on page 133).

SAFE SLEEPING

Reducing the risk of cot death

Sadly, we don't know why some babies die suddenly and for no apparent reason from what is called 'cot death' or 'Sudden Infant Death Syndrome' (SIDS). But we do know that placing a baby to sleep on his or her back reduces the risk, and that exposing a baby to cigarette smoke or overheating a baby increases the risk.

All the advice that we now have for reducing the risk of cot death and other dangers such as suffocation is listed below.

- **Always put your baby to sleep on his or her back.**

- **Cut out smoking in pregnancy – fathers too!**

- **Don't let anyone smoke in the same room as your baby.**

- **Don't let anyone have contact with your baby if they have smoked in the last 30-60 minutes as smoke is present in the expired air.**

- **Don't let your baby get too hot and don't overheat the room (see 'The right temperature', on the right).**

- **Keep your baby's head uncovered in bed – place your baby in the 'feet to foot' position (see picture).**

- **If your baby is unwell, seek advice promptly (see page 82).**

A safe place to sleep

- Your baby should always be put to sleep on his or her back unless there's clear medical advice to do something different. Babies sleeping on their backs *aren't* more likely to choke, and the risk of cot death is increased for babies sleeping on their fronts.

- It is advisable to keep your baby in a cot beside you for the first six months.

- Avoid plastic sheets or bumpers, ribbons and bits of string from mobiles. If they're anywhere near your baby, he or she could get tangled in them.

- Make sure there's no gap between the cot mattress and the sides of the cot through which your baby's body could slip. This is particularly important if you replace the mattress with a new or secondhand one. **If you do use a secondhand mattress, make sure that it is firm, clean and dry, well aired and generally in good condition.**

- Remove any loose plastic covering from the mattress that could come off and smother your baby.

- Don't give a baby under the age of one a pillow.

- Don't let anyone fall asleep nursing a baby.

- Don't let your baby fall asleep propped up on a cushion on a sofa or armchair.

The right temperature

Small babies aren't very good at controlling their own temperature. It's just as important to avoid them getting too hot as it is to avoid getting chilled. Overheating is known to be a factor in cot death.

- If the room is warm enough for you to be comfortable wearing light clothing (16–20°C), then it's the right temperature for your baby.

- Give your baby one light layer of clothing (or bedding) more than you're wearing. If the room is hot for you, keep your baby's clothes or bed covering light.

- Don't use duvets (quilts) until your baby is one year old. They get too hot.

- Although it is fine to take your baby into your bed for comfort, a baby falling asleep under your duvet may get too hot.

- Keep your baby's head uncovered indoors (unless it's very cold) because a baby needs to lose heat from his or her head and face.

- Never use a hot water bottle or electric blanket. Babies have a delicate skin, which can scald, or burn, easily.

- Ill or feverish babies don't need any extra bedding. In fact they usually need less.

- If you smoke, sharing a bed with your baby may increase the risk of cot death.

- Remove hats and extra clothing as soon as you come indoors or enter a warm car, bus or train, even if it means waking your baby.

Clean air
Babies shouldn't be exposed to tobacco smoke, either before birth or afterwards. If you, or anyone else who looks after your baby, smokes then don't smoke anywhere near the baby. It would be even better if everyone could make an effort to give up completely. Smoke is present in the air that is breathed out for a considerable time after smoking has taken place. Babies and young children who breathe in cigarette smoke are more likely to get coughs, asthma attacks, and chest and ear infections. For more on smoking see page 116.

Cot mattresses
Current research has found that there is absolutely no risk of cot death from toxic gases from fire-retardant materials found in some cot mattresses.

Following the advice given above will help reduce the risk of cot death.

BABIES WITH JAUNDICE AFTER TWO WEEKS

Many babies are jaundiced – which means they have yellow skin and eyes – for up to two weeks following birth. This is common in breastfed babies and usually does no harm. This is not a reason to stop breastfeeding. But, it is important to ensure that all is well if your baby is still jaundiced **after** two weeks. You should see your doctor within a day or two and this is particularly important if your baby's stools are pale or the urine is dark orange. Your doctor will arrange any tests that might be needed.

VITAMIN K

We all need vitamin K to make our blood clot properly so that we won't bleed too easily. Some newborn babies have too little vitamin K. Although this is rare, it can cause them to bleed dangerously. This is called 'haemorrhagic disease of the newborn'. To reduce the risk, you should be offered vitamin K which will be given to your baby. Your doctor or midwife will be able to explain these options and help you choose the method you prefer.

CRYING

A lot of people seem to think that babies shouldn't cry. They think that, if babies do cry, there must be a reason and you, the parent, should be able to do something about it. But all babies cry, and some cry a lot. Sometimes you'll know the reason. Often you'll try everything to stop it – change nappies, feed, rock, play – and yet nothing seems to work.

Here are some things you can try.

- **Let your baby suckle at your breast.**

- **Hold your baby close,** rocking, swaying, talking, singing. Or put your baby in a sling, held close against you. Move gently about, sway, and dance.

- **Rock your baby** backwards and forwards in the pram, or go out for a walk or a drive. Quite a lot of babies sleep in cars and even if your baby wakes up again the minute you stop, you've at least had a break.

- **Find things to look at or listen to** – music on the radio or a tape, a rattle, a mobile above the cot.

- **If your baby is bottle fed you can give him or her a dummy,** sterilised for small babies, never sweetened. Some babies find their thumb instead. Later, some will use a bit of cloth as a comforter; you can wash this as often as you need.

- **Stroke your baby** firmly and rhythmically holding him or her against you or lying face downwards on your lap. Or undress your baby and massage with baby oil, gently and firmly. Talk soothingly as you do it. Make sure the room is warm enough. Some clinics run courses to teach mothers baby massage - ask your midwife or health visitor about this.

- **Give your baby a warm bath.** This calms some babies instantly, but makes others cry even more. Like everything else, it might be worth a try.

- **Quietly put your baby down after a feed and leave the room for a few minutes.** Sometimes all the rocking and singing succeeds only in keeping your baby awake.

Remember
- **This difficult time won't last forever.** Your baby will gradually start to take more interest in the things around him or her and the miserable, frustrated crying will almost certainly stop.

- **Never shake your baby. Shaking makes a baby's or infant's head move violently. It causes bleeding and can damage the brain.** Sometimes you will feel very tired and even desperate. You might feel that you are losing control and have an urge to shake your baby But don't, this is dangerous.

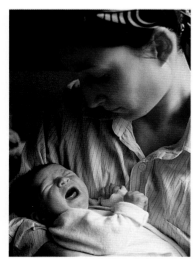

A WARNING CRY

Although all babies cry sometimes, there are times when crying may be a sign of illness. Watch out for a sudden change in the pattern or sound of your baby's crying. Often there may be a simple explanation: if you've been socialising more than usual your baby might simply be overtired and fretful. But if you feel that something is wrong, follow your feelings and contact your GP. See page 81 for more on what to do if you think your baby is ill.

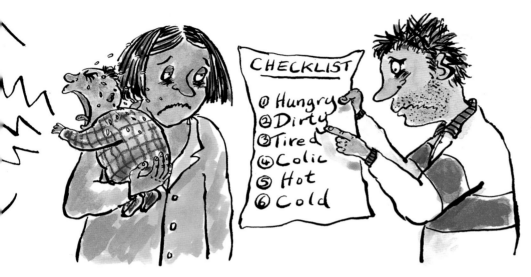

CHECKLIST
① Hungry
② Dirty
③ Tired
④ Colic
⑤ Hot
⑥ Cold

'At first it really upset me. I felt I ought to be able to comfort him, I ought to be able to make him happy, and he wasn't happy, and I couldn't comfort him, no matter what I did. And then it went on so long, it felt like forever, and I was still upset but I got sort of worn out by it, almost angry, because I was so disappointed that things weren't like I wanted them to be. I wanted to enjoy him, and I wanted him to be like other babies, smiling, gurgling, all of that, and he was just dreadful with the crying.'

Put your baby down safely in the cot or pram and calm yourself; don't be angry with your baby.

If you're finding it hard to cope you may need some help or support. Look on page 117 for suggestions. You could also ask for help from a friend, your health visitor or doctor. Or contact Serene (formerly known as CRY-SIS) (see page 133) who will put you in touch with other parents who've been in the same situation.

COLIC

Many babies have particular times in the day when they cry and cry and are difficult to comfort. Early evening is the usual bad patch. This is hard on you since it's probably the time when you are most tired and least able to cope.

Crying like this can be due to colic. Everybody agrees that colic exists, but there's disagreement about what causes it or even if there is always a cause. Some doctors say that it's a kind of stomach cramp, and it does seem to cause the kind of crying that might go with waves of

stomach pain – very miserable and distressed, stopping for a moment or two, then starting up again. The crying can go on for some hours, and there may be little you can do except try to comfort your baby and wait for the crying to pass. However, the following tips may help.

● **Try holding your baby in a way that puts gentle pressure and warmth on his or her stomach.** Try face down across your lap, or against your shoulder. Rhythmically rub and stroke your baby's back.

● **If you bottle feed your baby** and are worried that the milk doesn't agree with the baby, talk to your health visitor or doctor.

● **If you're breastfeeding,** it may be that something in your diet is upsetting your baby. When your baby seems colicky and uncomfortable, it may be worth looking back over what you've eaten in the last 24 hours. Make a note and discuss it with your health visitor, who may advise cutting out some foods for a while. Sometimes colic can also be a sign of too

'It was every evening. We'd be there, rocking her and walking up and down. We got so exhausted we were desperate. And then it stopped, gradually. You don't think you can bear it, but you do bear it, because there's nothing else for it. And in the end, it stops.'

'At some points I just didn't want to be involved at all. The first few months it was so much of a shock…I think that first bit – the sleepless broken nights and constant crying – I just couldn't handle it. I could quite easily have left it all to her, but then gradually I got used to it and you start to bond with the baby.'

(A FATHER)

23

THINGS TO ASK YOUR GP OR HEALTH VISITOR

Make a list of the questions you want to ask your GP or health visitor so you won't forget anything. It can help if you keep a record of how often and when your baby cries – for example, after every feed or during the evening. This may help you to identify the times when you need extra support or to see if a change of routine could help. For example, if your baby cries more in the afternoon and you go out in the morning, taking him or her out in the afternoon may be better. Or it may help the GP or health visitor to diagnose the problem. You might want to ask:

- *Is my baby physically well?*

- *(If you breastfeed) Should I change my diet?*

- *Is there any medication that could help?*

much fore milk. If your baby wakes up and cries up to half an hour following a breastfeed, try putting him or her back on to the breast he or she last fed from.

Coping with a colicky baby is extremely stressful. It may be best to tell yourself that there's nothing very much you can do. You just need to hang on as best you can until this part of your baby's life is over, which will certainly be only a few weeks. Just knowing that you're not causing the crying, and you can't do much to prevent it, may make it easier for you to bear. Try to take some time out for yourself whenever you can – maybe just handing over to someone else so that you can have a long, hot soak in the bath in the evening. Make sure that you get a decent meal every day to keep up your energy. If a crying baby occupies all your evening, then make lunch your main meal.

If the strain gets too much
- There may well be times when you're so tired you feel desperate, angry and can't take any more. Don't be ashamed to ask for help.

- **Try to share the crying times.** Think about handing your baby over to someone else for an hour. Nobody can cope alone with a constantly crying baby. You need someone who'll give you a break, at least occasionally, to calm down and get some rest.

- **Think about putting your baby down in the cot or pram and going away for a while.** Make sure your baby is safe, close the door, go into another room, and do what you can to calm yourself

down. Set a time limit – say, ten minutes – then go back.

- **Ask your health visitor if there is any local support for parents of crying babies.** Some areas run a telephone helpline. An organisation called Serene (formerly known as CRY-SIS) has branches in many areas and offers support through mothers who have had crying babies themselves. See page 133 for details of this and other support organisations.

Other remedies
- Some parents find giving their baby colic drops or gripe water helps. Others find these remedies are ineffective.

- Try massaging your baby's tummy in a clockwise direction with one drop of pure lavender oil to 10 mls of oil such as baby, soya or olive oil. (Avoid using almond or peanut oil if there are allergies in the family.)

- A drop of lavender oil placed on a cotton wool ball on a warm radiator or in a vaporiser may also soothe your baby.

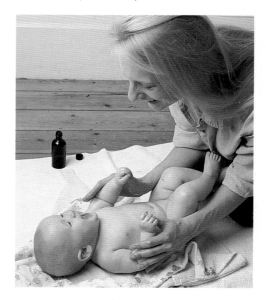

NAPPIES

WHAT'S IN A NAPPY?

Your baby's stools will be sticky and greenish/black at first (called 'meconium'). They will then change to a yellow or mustard colour which do not smell in a breastfed baby. Stools of a bottle-fed baby are darker brown and more smelly. Some infant formulas can also make the motions dark green. Breastfed babies have quite runny stools. Bottle-fed babies' stools are firmer. If you change from breast to bottle feeding you will find the stools become darker and more paste-like.

Some babies fill their nappies at or around every feed. Some, especially breastfed babies, can go for several days, even a week, without a bowel movement. Both are quite normal. It is usual for babies to strain or even cry when passing a stool. Your baby is not constipated if the stools are soft.

From day to day or week to week, your baby's stools will probably vary a bit. But if you notice a marked change of any kind, such as the stools becoming any of the following – very smelly, very watery, very pale (see page 21 for information on jaundice), or becoming hard, particularly if there's blood in them – you should talk to your doctor or health visitor.

NAPPY CHANGING

Some babies have very delicate skin and need changing the minute they wet themselves if they're not to get sore and red. Others seem to be tougher and get along fine with a change before or after every feed. All babies need to be changed when they're dirty to prevent nappy rash and because they can smell awful!

NAPPY RASH

Most babies get nappy rash at some time in the first 18 months. This is most commonly caused by the skin being in prolonged contact with ammonia from urine or bacteria from stools burning or irritating the skin, which may then break open. Other causes include:

- *a sensitive skin*
- *rubbing or chaffing*
- *strong soap, detergent or bubble bath*
- *baby wipes containing alcohol*
- *diarrhoea or illnesses*
- *changes in diet such as weaning or changing from breast milk to formula.*

In its early stages the rash may appear as red patches on your baby's bottom or there may be general redness. The skin may look sore and be hot to touch and there may be spots, pimples or blisters.

Getting organised

- Get everything you need for changing in one place before you start. The best place to change a nappy is on a changing mat or towel on the floor, particularly if you've more than one baby. If you sit down you won't hurt your back and, as your baby gets bigger, he or she can't wriggle off and hurt him or herself. If you're using a changing table, keep one hand on your baby at all times.

- Make sure you've a supply of nappies. If you're using terries, ask a friend or your midwife to show you how to fold and pin them. Experiment to find out what suits you best.

- You'll need a supply of cotton wool and a bowl of warm water or baby lotion, or baby wipes.

- Make sure you've a spare set of clothes. In the early weeks you often need to change everything.

TO PROTECT YOUR BABY AGAINST NAPPY RASH

- *Change the nappy as soon as you can when it becomes wet or soiled. You may find your young baby needs changing 10 to 12 times a day, and older children at least 6 to 8 times.*

- *Clean the whole nappy area thoroughly, wiping from front to back. Use a mild baby soap with plain water, or specially formulated baby lotion or gentle baby wipes. If using soap and water, rinse off the soap and pat dry thoroughly and gently.*

- *Lie your baby on a towel and leave the nappy off for as long and as often as you can to let fresh air get to the skin.*

TO TREAT NAPPY RASH:

Follow the steps outlined in '*To protect your baby against nappy rash*' on page 25 and also:

- *Apply a nappy rash cream to help healing – ask your health visitor or pharmacist to recommend one.*

- *If the rash does not go away after treatment or there is a persistent bright-red moist rash with white or red pimples, which also affects the folds of the skin, this may be due to a thrush infection. In this case, a special anti-fungal cream available from your pharmacist or on prescription from your doctor, will be needed.*

NAPPY SERVICES

If you use disposable nappies, it is worth enquiring whether any shop in your area provides a free delivery service. Or, if you use terry nappies, you may be able to use a nappy laundering service.

Getting started

- If your baby is dirty, use the nappy to clean off most of it. Then, using the cotton wool, a mild baby soap and warm water, baby lotion or gentle baby wipes, clean girls from front to back to avoid getting germs into the vagina. Boys should be cleaned around the penis and testicles (balls). Don't pull back the foreskin when cleaning the penis. It's just as important to clean carefully when you're changing a wet nappy.

- You can use a barrier cream, which helps to protect against nappy rash, but it's usually enough just to leave your baby's skin clean and dry. Some babies are sensitive to these creams and some thick creams may clog nappies or affect the ability of disposable nappies to absorb wetness.

- Avoid using baby powder because it can make your baby choke.

- If you're using a terry nappy, fold it, put in a nappy liner if you wish, pin it with a proper nappy pin that won't spring open, and put on or tie on plastic pants.

- If you're using disposable nappies, take care not to get water or cream on the sticky tabs as they won't stick. You can now buy extra tabs to stick disposable nappies (or sticky tape will do).

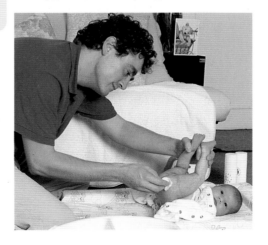

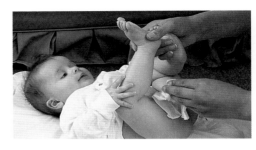

NAPPY HYGIENE

Put as much of the contents as you can down the toilet. If you're using terries with disposable liners the liner can be flushed away, but don't ever flush a nappy down the toilet because you'll block it.

Disposable nappies can be rolled up and resealed with the tabs. Put them in a plastic bag kept only for nappies, then tie it up and place it in an outside bin.

Terries must be washed and sterilised. You'll need a plastic bucket with a lid, which must be refilled every day with clean water and sterilising powder made up to the manufacturer's instructions. Each nappy must be soaked in the steriliser following the instructions and then a load can be washed every day. Use very hot water and avoid enzyme (bio) washing powders and fabric conditioners, which can irritate your baby's skin. Make sure the nappies are very well rinsed.

Remember to wash your hands after changing a nappy and before doing anything else in order to avoid infection. It's worth remembering that the polio virus is passed in a baby's stools for a month after each polio immunisation. Tell your childminder or babysitter, or anyone else who is likely to change nappies during this time, to be extra careful about washing their hands after changing the nappy and disposing of its contents as there is a very small risk of the virus causing polio in an unimmunised person. They may wish to have a polio booster themselves.

WASHING AND BATHING

WASHING

Wash your baby's face, neck, hands and bottom carefully every day. This is often called 'topping and tailing'. Choose a time when your baby is awake and contented and make sure the room is warm. Organise everything you need in advance – a bowl of warm water, a towel, cotton wool, a fresh nappy and, if necessary, clean clothes.

- Hold your baby on your knee, or lie your baby on a changing mat, and take off all your baby's clothes except for a vest and nappy. Then wrap your baby in the towel.

- Dip the cotton wool in the water (not too much) and wipe gently around your baby's eyes from the nose outward, using a fresh piece of cotton wool for each eye.

- Using a fresh piece of cotton wool, clean around your baby's ears, but don't clean inside them.

- Wash the rest of your baby's face, neck and hands in the same way and dry them gently with the towel.

- Now change your baby's nappy as described on page 25.

In the first ten days you should also clean around your baby's navel each day. Your midwife will show you how.

BATHING

Bathing two or three times a week is quite enough, but you can do it daily if your baby enjoys it. Don't bath your baby straight after a feed or when your baby is hungry or tired. Make sure the room is warm.

Have everything you need at hand – a baby bath or washing up bowl filled with warm water, two towels (in case of accidents!), baby bath liquid (but avoid this if your baby has particularly dry skin) or baby soap, a clean nappy, clean clothes and cotton wool.

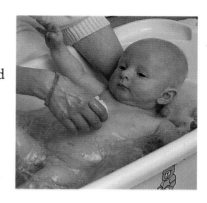

- Make sure the water is warm, *not* hot; check it with your wrist or elbow.

- Hold your baby on your knee and follow the instructions given above for cleaning his or her face.

- Wash your baby's hair with baby soap or liquid, then rinse carefully, supporting your baby over the bowl. Dry gently.

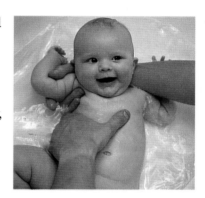

- Now remove your baby's nappy, wiping away any mess. If you're using baby soap, soap your baby all over (avoiding his or her face) while still on your knee, keeping a firm grip while you do so.

- Lower your baby gently into the bowl using one hand to hold your baby's upper arm and support his or her head and shoulders; keep your baby's head clear of the water. Use the other hand to gently swish the water over your baby without splashing. *Never* **leave your baby alone in the bath;** not even for a second.

- Lift your baby out and pat dry, paying special attention to the creases. You may want to use this time to massage baby oil into your baby's skin. Many babies love this and it may help your baby relax and sleep. Lay your baby on a towel on the floor as both the baby – and your hands – might be a bit slippery.

If your baby seems frightened of bathing and cries, you could try bathing together, but make sure the water is not too hot. It's easier if someone else holds your baby while you get in and out.

TAKING YOUR BABY OUT

Your baby is ready to go out as soon as you feel fit enough to go yourself.

WALKING

Walking is good for both of you. It may be easiest to take a tiny baby in a sling. If you use a buggy make sure your baby can lie down with his or her back flat.

IN A CAR

It's illegal for anyone to hold a baby while sitting in the front seat of a car. The only safe way for your baby to travel in a car is in a properly secured, backward-facing, baby seat, or in a carrycot (not a Moses basket) with the cover on and secured with special straps.

If you have a car with air bags in the front your baby should **not** travel in the front seat (even facing backwards) because of the danger of suffocation if the bag inflates.

Some areas have special loan schemes to enable you to borrow a suitable baby seat when you and your baby first return from hospital. Ask your midwife or health visitor.

IN COLD WEATHER

Make sure your baby is wrapped up warm in cold weather because babies chill very easily. **Take the extra clothing off when you get into a warm place** so that your baby doesn't then overheat, even if he or she is asleep.

IN HOT WEATHER

Children are particularly vulnerable to the effects of the sun, as their skin is thinner and they may not be able to produce enough pigment called melanin to protect them from sunburn. Children with fair or red hair, blue eyes and freckles are especially at risk, as the paler the skin, the less melanin is produced, and the more likely the child is to get burnt in the sun. Keep babies under six months out of the sun altogether. Older children should always be protected, either by covering them up or with a high protection sunscreen (sun protection factor 15+). Babies' and children's skin burn easily, even in sun which wouldn't affect your own skin. See page 104 for further tips on protecting your child from the sun.

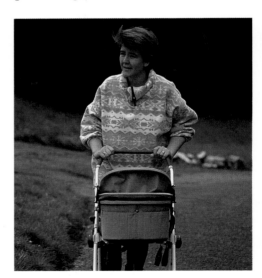

TWINS (OR MORE)

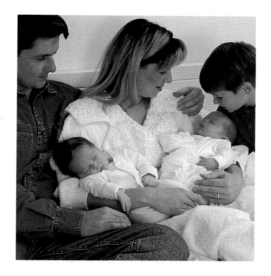

Parents with only one child often think that having two together is much the same sort of experience, but doubled. If you have twins, you'll know differently. Caring for twins, or more, is very different from caring for two of different ages. There's certainly a lot more work, and often you need to find different ways of doing things.

You need as much support as you can get. If you've more than two babies you may be able to get a home help from your local council. Find out what their policy is. A few hours of help with housework a week could make a big difference. If your council doesn't provide home helps, ask your health visitor for any suggestions. The Multiple Births Foundation also offers professional support and a range of direct services to families of twins and other multiple births (address on page 136).

You may get a lot of help from family and friends, but it also helps to be in contact with other parents of twins. The Twins and Multiple Births Association (TAMBA; address on page 136) offers a lot of helpful information, including information about local Twins Clubs. Through these clubs you can meet other parents whose experiences are like yours, and get support and practical advice. Often you can get secondhand equipment too, such as twin prams and buggies.

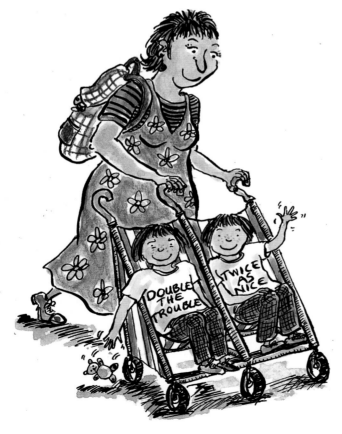

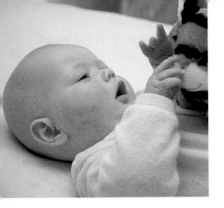

2 How your child will grow

Your baby may walk at 11 months. Your neighbour's baby may still be crawling at 16 months. Both are quite normal. One child may be talking in sentences at two years old, another may have just started to put two words together. Both are normal. Each child is different because each is an individual. This chapter looks at the way children grow.

HOW CHILDREN DEVELOP

'When he does something new that he's never done before, that's magic. It's like no other baby in the world has ever done it.'

(A FATHER)

'My mum said, "Isn't she walking yet?" And as it happened, the little boy next door who's about the same age was up and walking and Annie was just sitting there not doing a thing. My mum said I was walking at that age. She kept going on about it.'

'I want to know that she's all right and, you know, keeping up.'

(A FATHER)

Children aren't just born different, they also have different lives and they'll learn different things. A child who plays a lot with toys will be learning to use his or her hands and eyes together. A child who goes out to the park every day will soon learn the names of ducks and trees. A child who is often talked to will learn more words. A child who's given love and praise for learning new things will want to learn more.

Some children have difficulty learning, perhaps because of physical problems with, for example, hearing or seeing. You may already know that your child's development is likely to be slower than normal or you may be worried about your child's progress. Your child may be offered regular development reviews (see page 36) but you don't have to wait for a checkup. If you're concerned, talk to your health visitor or GP. If something's holding your child back, the sooner you find out, the sooner you can do something to help. For more on this see page 40. For more about play and learning see pages 41–47.

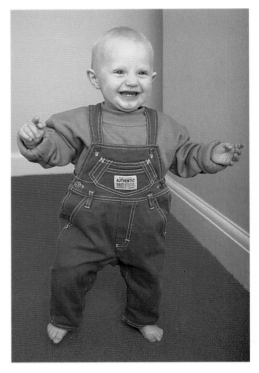

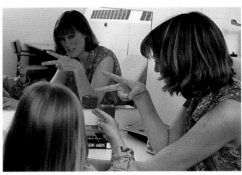

FEET – AND FIRST SHOES

Babies' and small children's feet grow very fast and it's important that the bones grow straight.

- The bones in a baby's toes are soft at birth. If they're cramped by tight bootees, socks, stretch suits or pram shoes, the toes can't straighten out and grow properly. So keep your baby's feet as free as possible. Make sure bootees and socks leave room for their toes, both in length and width. If the feet of a stretch suit become too small, cut them off and use socks instead.

- Don't put your child into proper shoes until he or she can walk alone, and keep them only for walking outside at first.

- When you buy shoes, always have your child's feet measured by a qualified fitter. Shoes should be about 1 cm (a bit less than ½ in) beyond the longest toe and wide enough for all the toes to lie flat.

- Shoes with a lace, buckle or velcro fastening hold the heel in place and stop the foot slipping forward and damaging the toes. If the heel of a shoe slips off when your child stands on tiptoe, it doesn't fit.

- It's better to buy cheaper shoes made of cotton or canvas and throw them away as soon as they're worn out, than expensive ones that you can't afford to replace often enough. Have your child's feet measured for each new pair.

- Check that socks are the right size and discard any outgrown or misshapen socks. Cotton ones are best.

- Don't keep shoes for 'best' as your child may outgrow these without having proper wear.

- Buy footwear made of natural materials, i.e. leather, cotton or canvas as these materials 'breathe'. Plastic shoes make feet perspire and may cause fungal infections and abrasions.

COMMON FOOT PROBLEMS

When children first start walking it is normal for them to walk with their feet apart and to 'waddle'. It is also common for young children to appear to be 'bow-legged', 'knock-kneed' or walk with their toes turned in or out. Most minor foot problems in children correct themselves. But if you are worried about your child's feet or how he or she walks in any way, talk to your doctor or health visitor. If necessary, your child can be referred to a chiropodist, orthopaedic surgeon or paediatric physiotherapist.

- ***Bow legs*** *– a small gap between the knees and ankles when the child is standing up is normally seen until the child is two. If the gap is pronounced or it does not correct itself, check with your doctor or health visitor. Rarely, this could be a sign of rickets – a bone deformity.*

- ***Knock knees*** *– this is when a child stands with his or her knees together and the ankles are at least 2.5 cm (1 in) apart. Between the ages of two and four, a gap of 6 to 7 cm is considered normal. Knock knees usually improve and correct themselves by the age of six.*

- ***In-toeing*** *(pigeon-toed) – here the child's feet turn in. The condition usually corrects itself by the age of eight or nine and treatment is not usually needed.*

- ***Out-toeing*** *(feet point outwards) – again this condition usually corrects itself and treatment is not needed in most cases.*

- ***Flat feet*** *– if when your child stands on tip-toe the arch forms normally, no treatment is needed.*

- ***Tiptoe walking*** *– if your child walks on tiptoes, talk to your doctor or health visitor.*

A GUIDE TO DEVELOPMENT

This guide gives an idea of the age range within which most children gain certain skills. The ages given are averages. Lots of perfectly normal children gain one skill earlier, another later than average. You can tick off each thing as your child achieves a new skill and keep it as a record for development reviews (see page 36)

YEARS 1 2 3 4 5
MONTHS 1 2 3 4 5 6 7 8 9 10 11 12 13 14 15 16 17 18 24 36 48 60

MOVEMENT

Lift their heads, while lying on their fronts.

Sit without support. If your baby is not sitting unsupported by nine months, talk to your health visitor or GP.

Start trying to crawl. Some babies crawl backwards before they crawl forwards. Some learn to walk without ever crawling. Others are bottom shufflers.

Pull themselves upright and stand, holding on to the furniture.

Walk alone. If your child is not walking by 18 months, talk to your health visitor or GP.

Learn to kick or throw a ball. Throwing sometimes takes longer than kicking.

HANDLING THINGS

Reach out for objects.

Can hold an object and will lift it up to suck it. At first, babies can hold objects, but are unable to let go.

Learn to pass things from hand to hand.

Learn to let go of things, for example, to drop something or give it to you.

Feed themselves 'finger foods'.

Begin to feed themselves very messily, with a spoon and to take off easily removed clothes (like loose, short socks).

Begin to build with bricks. Large bricks are easiest to start with.

Enjoy scribbling with a crayon.

Can draw what you see is a person (with a face and maybe arms and legs). Like much else, this depends a lot on how much practice and encouragement they get.

Can use a knife and fork.

HEARING AND TALKING

Startled by sudden, loud noises.

By 4 months: Make cooing noises, like 'gagaga...' and enjoy making more and more different sounds.

By 6 months: make repetitive noises, like 'gagaga...' and enjoy making more and more different sounds.

By 7 months: Turn to your voice across the room, or to very quiet noises on either side if not distracted by something else.

By 12 months: Respond to their own name, say something like 'mama' and 'dada', to parents.

By 18 months: Can say between 6 and 20 recognisable words, but understand many more. They also start to use language in play, for example when feeding a teddy or doll, or talking on a toy telephone.

By 2 years: Can put at least two words together and can point to parts of their body.

By 3-3½ years: Can talk well in sentences, chant rhymes and songs, and talk clearly enough to be understood by strangers. A few 3-year-olds may be difficult to understand. It's normal for a 2-year-old to pronounce words incorrectly. If your 3-year old is hard to understand mention this to your health visitor.

SEEING

In the first few weeks: especially like looking at faces. Babies will focus on a face close in front of them, and follow it.

By 2 weeks: Begin to recognise their parents.

By 4-6 weeks: May start to smile.

By 6 weeks: Can follow a brightly coloured moving toy, held about 20 cm (8in) away.

By 6 months: Can see across a room.

- Walk out of any shop that asks you the size of your child's feet and does not measure them.

- Never rely on the question 'do they feel comfortable?' Because children's bones are soft, distortion and cramping can be present without your child feeling it.

- Children under four years old should have their feet measured every 6 to 8 weeks, and over four, every 10 to 12 weeks.

- Never buy secondhand shoes or hand shoes down as these take on the shape of the previous owner and will rub and not support vital areas.

- After washing your child's feet, dry well between the toes, and cut toenails straight across – they can become ingrown if cut shaped.

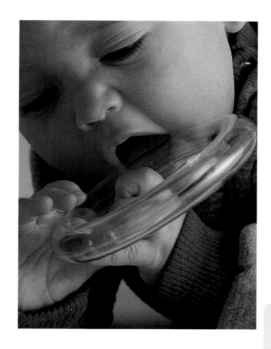

TEETH

The time when babies get their first primary teeth (milk teeth) varies. A few are born with a tooth already through. Others have no teeth at one year old. Most get their first tooth at around six months, usually in front and at the bottom. Most have all their primary teeth by about two and a half. The first permanent 'second' teeth come through at the back at around the age of six.

There are 20 primary teeth in all, 10 at the top and 10 at the bottom.

TEETHING

Some teeth come through with no pain or trouble at all. At other times you may notice that the gum is sore and red where the tooth is coming, or that one cheek is flushed. Your baby may dribble, gnaw and chew a lot, or just be fretful, but it's often hard to tell whether this is really due to teething.

It can help to give your baby something hard to chew on such as a teething ring, or a dried crust of bread, or a peeled carrot **(stay nearby in case of choking)**. Avoid rusks because almost all contain some sugar. Constant chewing and sucking on sugary things can cause tooth decay, even if your baby has only one or two teeth.

For babies over four months old you can try sugar-free teething gel rubbed on the gum. You can get this from the pharmacist. For younger babies you should talk to your GP or health visitor. You may also want to give sugar-free baby paracetamol. Follow the instructions on the bottle for your child's age, or check with your pharmacist, GP or health visitor.

People put all sorts of things down to teething – rashes, crying, bad temper, runny noses, extra dirty nappies. But be careful not to explain away what might be the signs of illness by saying it's 'just teething'.

FLUORIDE

Fluoride is a natural element found in our diet, mostly in fish and tea, which can help prevent tooth decay. It is also present in many water supplies, but usually at a level too low to be beneficial. In the UK, Birmingham and Newcastle have fluoride added to the water supply at the ideal level, as do most cities in the USA.

In areas with little or no fluoride in the water, some children may benefit by taking fluoride drops (for babies) or tablets as dietary supplements. They should not be used in areas with fluoride naturally present or artificially added to the water, as an excessive fluoride intake is undesirable. Therefore advice from your dentist, is essential before giving them. Fluoride in toothpaste is very effective – for babies use a tiny smear and for children only use a small pea-sized amount on the brush.

LOOKING FOR SUGARS ON THE LABEL

- *The following are sugars that can cause dental decay – sucrose, glucose, dextrose, maltose, fructose, hydrolysed starch.*

- *Invert sugar or syrup, honey, raw sugar, brown sugar, cane sugar, muscavado and concentrated fruit juices all contain sugars.*

- *Fruit juices contain sugars, which can cause decay too. Always dilute these.*

- *Maltodextrin is not a sugar, but may cause decay.*

CARING FOR YOUR CHILD'S TEETH

- Keep down the number of times each day that your child eats or drinks something sugary.

- Brush your child's teeth thoroughly, twice each day, using a small pea-sized amount of fluoride toothpaste or a tiny smear for babies; help an older child. Let your child see you brushing your teeth too.

Cutting down on sugar

Sugar causes tooth decay. It's not just the amount of sugar in sweet food and drinks that matters but, perhaps more importantly, how often there are sugary things in the mouth. This is why sweet drinks in a bottle and lollipops are so bad. The teeth are bathed in sugar for quite a long time.

- **From the time you start your baby on foods and drinks other than milk, avoid giving sweet things.** Try to encourage savoury tastes. Watch for the sugar in baby foods in tins and packets (even the savoury varieties), and rusks and in baby drinks, especially fizzy drinks, squash and syrups.

- **If you give your child sweet foods and fruit juice try to limit these to mealtimes** to avoid tooth decay. Well diluted fruit juice containing vitamin C and given with a meal, in a cup, can also help iron to be absorbed. Between meals, it is better to give milk or water as a drink.

- **Try to find treats other than biscuits or sweets,** and ask relatives and friends to do the same. Use things like stickers, badges, hair slides, crayons, small books, notebooks and colouring books, soap and bubble baths.

These may be more expensive than one small sweet, but they all last longer.

- **If children are given sweets or chocolate, it's less harmful for their teeth if they eat them all at once and after a meal,** than if they eat, say, a little every hour or so.

- Children who eat sweets every day have nearly double the decay compared to children who eat sweets less often.

- **Be aware of the amount of sugar the whole family's eating.** Look for ways of cutting down. See pages 76–77 for some suggestions.

- **Avoid giving baby juices or sugar-sweetened drinks at bedtime** or in a bottle, and keep drinking times short. Only milk or water should be given as a drink during the night (unless your baby is still young enough to need a night feed).

- **Ask your pharmacist and doctor for sugar-free medicine** for your child.

- **Don't give too many drinks containing the artificial sweetener saccharin. If you do, dilute with at least 10 parts water to 1 part concentrate.**

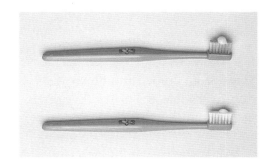

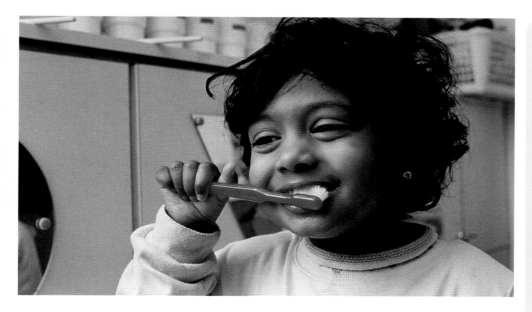

BRUSHING YOUR CHILD'S TEETH

- **Start early, as soon as your baby's teeth start to come through.** Buy a baby toothbrush and use it with a tiny smear of fluoride toothpaste. Check with your dentist whether baby toothpaste has enough fluoride for your baby's needs. Don't worry if you don't manage to brush much at first. The important thing at the start is to get teeth brushing accepted as part of the everyday routine. That's why it's important you do it too.

- **Gradually start to brush your child's teeth more thoroughly, brushing all the surfaces of the teeth.** Do it twice a day – just before bed, and whatever other time in the day fits in best. Not all children like having their teeth brushed, so you may have to work at it a bit. Try not to let it become a battle. If it becomes difficult, try games, or try brushing your own teeth at the same time and then helping your child to 'finish off'.

- **Go on helping your child to brush until you're sure he or she is brushing well enough – at least until the age of 7.**

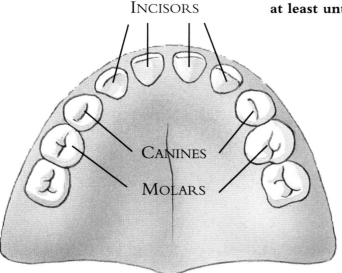

INCISORS

CANINES

MOLARS

HOW TO BRUSH

The best way to brush a baby's teeth is to sit him or her on your knee with the head resting against your chest. Stand behind an older child and tilt his or her head upwards. Brush the teeth in small circles covering all the surfaces and let your child spit the toothpaste out afterwards. Rinsing with water has been found to reduce the benefit of fluoride. You can also clean your baby's teeth by wrapping your finger over a piece of damp gauze with a tiny amount of fluoride toothpaste.

TAKING YOUR CHILD TO THE DENTIST

You can take your child to be registered with a dentist under the NHS as soon as your child has been born – even before any teeth come through. Your dentist can give advice on your child's oral health. NHS dental treatment for children is free.

Take your child with you when you go to the dentist, so that going to the dentist becomes a normal event. If you need to find a dentist, you can ask at your local clinic or contact your local health authority – the address and telephone number will be in the phone book.

KEEPING AN EYE ON YOUR BABY'S GROWTH AND DEVELOPMENT

PARENT-HELD RECORDS

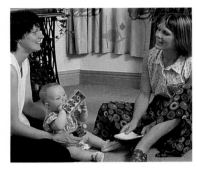

In most clinics now you'll be given a personal child health record or parent-held record for your baby. This is a way of keeping track of your child's progress. It makes sure that, wherever you are and whatever happens to your child, you'll have a copy of the records for your own information and for health professionals when and where you may need it.

To start with you'll want to use the records mainly to record your child's height and weight. Then you can add information about immunisations (see pages 94–101), childhood illness and accidents. These records are quite new and health visitors or doctors may not always remember to fill them in. It's important to remind them to do so, so that there's a full record of your child's health.

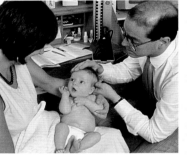

DEVELOPMENT REVIEWS

Your GP and health visitor will offer you regular development reviews. The review gives you, the parents, an opportunity to say what you've noticed about your child. You can also discuss anything at all that may concern you about your child's health and general behaviour. Not just the big things, but the kinds of worries and niggles that every parent has but feels unsure about taking to a doctor or nurse.

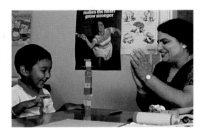

The review programme
Development reviews will usually be carried out by your health visitor, sometimes alone and sometimes with a doctor. They may be carried out at a regular clinic session or in your own home. The aim is to spot any problems as early as possible so that, if necessary, some action can be taken. So, even if you think your child is doing fine, it's worth having the review. Your health visitor will tell you when it's due but, if you're concerned about something at any other time, don't wait. Ask to see someone.

You can usually expect to be invited to a development review when your child is:

- 6 to 8 weeks old

- 6 to 9 months old

- 18 to 24 months old

- 3 to 3½ years old

- 4½ to 5½ years old (before or just after your child starts school).

In some parts of the country, the age that your child is reviewed may vary slightly to those given above, especially after the age of three.

HEIGHT AND WEIGHT

Your child's height and weight are a very useful guide to general progress and development. You can have your baby regularly weighed at your child health clinic or doctor's baby clinic. Older children should be weighed and measured as part of other health checks. Babies vary in how fast they put on weight, but usually weight gain is quickest in the first six to nine months, and then it slows down.

- Most babies double their birthweight by four to five months.

- Most babies treble their birthweight by one year.

Some weeks your baby will gain weight; some weeks he or she will not gain weight. This doesn't matter. What's looked for is a general weight gain over a period of weeks.

Understanding your child's height and weight chart

Your child's growth will be recorded on 'centile' charts so that his or her progress can be easily followed. Boys and girls have different charts because boys are on average heavier and taller and their growth pattern is slightly different. Page 38 shows an example of a boy's height weight and head size centile lines for babies up to one year old; this page shows a girl's height and weight centile lines for children from one to five.

The new charts were produced in 1996, based on the latest information about child growth and are always kept up-to-date.

The centile lines printed on the

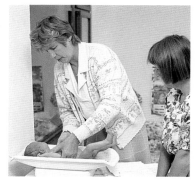

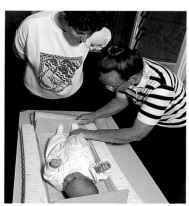

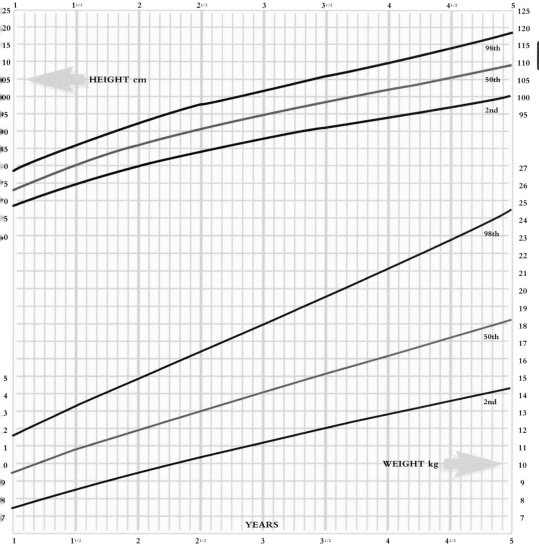

Girls | 1 to 5 years

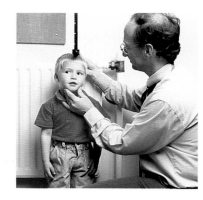

charts show roughly the kind of growth expected in weight and in length. On each of the charts the middle line (shown as a red line in this book) represents the national average for white British babies. For example, if 100 babies are weighed and measured, 50 will weigh and measure more than the amount indicated by the red line, and 50 will weigh and measure less.

Most babies' and children's weight and height will fall between the two centile lines coloured blue in this book. Only four out of every 100 babies and children will have weights and heights that fall outside these centiles.

As these data are based on the average heights and weights of white children, it's worth bearing in mind that if you're of Asian origin your baby will on average be lighter

and shorter. If you're of African-Caribbean origin your baby will on average be heavier and longer.

Your child's height and weight (and head size if under a year) will be plotted as a curved line on one of these charts. This makes it easy to see how your child is developing.

Whatever weight and length your baby is at birth, he or she should have a fairly steady growth, resulting in a line curving in roughly the same way, and usually inside, the centile lines on the chart.

During the first two years of life it is quite usual for a baby's line to cross the centiles on the chart from time to time, but if at any time your baby's weight line suddenly goes up or drops (and it may drop, for example, because of illness), talk to your health visitor or GP about it.

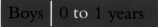

Boys | 0 to 1 years

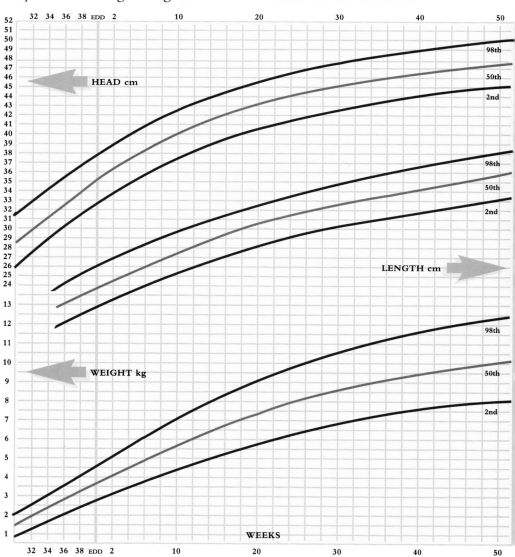

ou should also talk to your health
isitor or GP if, after the age of two,
our baby's height curve does not
ollow a centile line or starts to veer
pwards or downwards from it.

ENERAL DEVELOPMENT

ome health visitors may ask your
hild to do little tasks such as
uilding with blocks or identifying
ictures. Others may simply watch
our child playing or perhaps
rawing, and get an idea from this
bservation, and your comments, of
ow your child is doing. If you look
the development chart on page 32
ou'll have an idea of the kind of
hysical and verbal skills they're
oking for. If your child's first
anguage isn't English, you may need
ask if development reviews can be
rried out with the help of
meone who can speak your child's
anguage. See page 125 for
formation about linkworkers.

If your child seems slow in one
articular area of development you'll
ave the opportunity to discuss what
e reason may be. And to see
hether there's anything useful that
eeds to be done to speed things up.

YESIGHT

baby should be able to see from
rth. Eyesight develops gradually
ver the next six months.

By the first review, you'll have
oticed whether or not your baby
n follow a colourful object held
bout 20cms (8 inches) away with
s or her eyes. If this isn't happening
ou should mention it.

At birth a baby's eyes may roll
way from each other occasionally. If
baby is squinting all, or much, of
e time tell your health visitor and
our GP.

If your baby is squinting you'll
need to be referred to an orthoptist
or ophthalmologist who specialises
in understanding children's eyes.

HEARING AND TALKING

Hearing and talking are linked. If
your child can't hear properly he or
she will have great difficulty learning
to talk and may need to be taught
other ways of communicating. So
the sooner hearing problems are
discovered the greater the chance
that something can be done.

It isn't only hearing that is
important though. Babies don't learn
to talk unless they're talked to, even
if, at first, the conversation is limited
to making noises at each other. By
learning to take it in turns to make
babbling noises, your baby is
learning what a conversation feels
like. Most parents quite naturally
join in babbling sessions with their
babies and so they're very often the
first people to notice if there's a
problem.

If you're ever worried about your
child's language development, talk to
your GP or health visitor. Your child
may be helped by referral to a
speech and language therapist.

Your baby's hearing may be tested
at birth in the hospital. No baby is
'too young' for a hearing assessment.

You should expect a hearing
assessment at six to nine months. If
there's no apparent problem, but
you're still worried, ask for another
appointment. If a problem is found,
your baby will need to have a
follow-up assessment because
hearing loss may be temporary, due
to a cold or a passing infection.

If your child doesn't seem to hear
properly at the second appointment,
or you are still worried, ask for a
referral to a specialist.

*You may find that when
your child is reviewed, the
doctor or health visitor will
not formally 'test' your child
but will ask you questions
about what he or she can or
can't do. It is therefore
helpful if you record these
details in your child's
personal child health record
and complete the
questionnaires in the book
before your child has a
review. Don't forget to take
the book with you when you
take your child for a review!*

*Remember too that, even if
your child's development is
satisfactory at one review,
development is a continuous
process. It is therefore
important that you continue
to observe your child's
development, attend all the
reviews and talk to your
health visitor or GP if you
have any concerns about
your child between these
reviews.*

BILINGUAL CHILDREN

*Children who are growing
up in a family who speak
more than one language
don't usually have problems.
A few develop language
more slowly. The important
thing is to talk to your child
in whatever language feels
comfortable to you. This
may mean one parent using
one language and the other
using another. Children
usually adapt to this
very well.*

SOME QUESTIONS
YOU MAY LIKE TO ASK

CHILDREN WITH SPECIAL NEEDS

You may find it helpful to write these down.

- *Is there a name for my child's problem? If so, what is it?*
- *Are more tests needed to get a clear diagnosis or confirm what's been found out?*
- *Is it likely to get better or likely to get worse, or will it stay roughly the same?*
- *Where is the best place to go for medical help?*
- *Where is the best place to go for practical help?*
- *How can I get in touch with other parents who have children with a similar problem?*
- *How can I find out how best to help my child?*

COPING WITH YOUR FEELINGS

At whatever stage in your child's life you receive a diagnosis of disability or illness, you'll have difficult feelings to cope with, and some hard decisions and adjustments to make. Your GP, health visitor, social worker or counsellors of various kinds may all be able to help. So may other parents who've been through similar experiences. But, even with help, all parents say it takes time. Throughout that time, and afterwards, it's right to think about your own life and needs as well as your child's.

For some families, everything is not 'all right'. Sometimes what begins as a worry does turn out to be a more serious problem or disability.

If this happens to you, your first need will be for information about the problem and what it's likely to mean for your child and for you. You'll have a lot of questions (see box). Put them all to your GP, your health visitor and to specialists to whom you are referred. You may find it easier to make a list.

Be determined and persist if you need to. Not all health professionals talk easily or well to parents. And you yourself may find it's difficult to hear and take in all that's said to you first, or even second, time round. Rather than live with unanswered questions, go back and ask again for the information or opinion you feel you need. Or you could take along a tape recorder. If, in the end, the honest answer is 'I don't know' or 'We're not sure', that's better than no answer at all.

HELP FOR CHILDREN WITH SPECIAL NEEDS

Child development centres

In some areas, teams of professionals (doctors, therapists, health visitors, social workers), usually working from what is known as a child development centre, are available to help support children with special needs and their families. You can be referred to such a team through your GP or health visitor.

Voluntary organisations

You can also get information, advice and support from organisations dealing with particular handicaps, illnesses and other problems.

Through them, you can often contact other parents in situations like your own. See pages 133–36 for the names and addresses of some organisations that might be able to help.

Specialist help

There are many services available to help children who have special needs to learn and develop, for example, physiotherapy, speech and language therapy, occupational therapy, home learning schemes, playgroups, opportunity groups, nurseries and nursery schools and classes. To find out what's available in your area, ask your health visitor, GP, social services department or the educational adviser for special needs at your local education department. See pages 124–126 for more information about the services, including information about regional variations.

Special needs assessment

Local education authorities who think a child over two years old may have special educational needs *must* make an assessment of his or her needs. For a child under two an assessment must be made if a parent *asks* for it. This assessment is a way of getting advice about your child's educational needs. You can take part in the assessment yourself. The Advisory Centre for Education (see page 134) offers advice on education and produces a handbook on the subject.

Benefits advice

For information about social security benefits for children with special needs, see page 132. See also **Help with National Health Service costs** on page 131.

3 Learning and playing

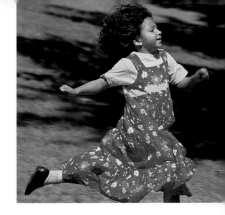

What we call playing is really the way children learn. With toys and their imaginations they practice all the skills they'll need as they grow up. The more they play, the more they learn and the best thing about it is that they love it.

PLAYING WITH YOU

Young children find it hard to play alone. They need attention from someone who can play with them. Gradually they'll learn to entertain themselves for some of the time, but first they need to learn how to do that.

In the meantime, you can't spend all your time playing. You've other things to do and other people to attend to. Fortunately, children learn from everything that's going on around them, and everything they do. When you're washing up, your toddler can stand next to you on a chair and wash the saucepan lids; when you cook, make sure your baby can see and talk to you as you work.

The times when they're not learning much are the times when they're bored. That's as true for babies as of older children. So what really matters?

- Find a lot of different things for your child to look at, think about, and do (see **Ideas for play** on pages 43-44).

- Make what you're doing fun and interesting for your child, so you can get it done.

- Make some time to give all your attention to what your child wants to do.

TOY SAFETY

- *It is best to buy toys that carry the British Standard kitemark or the Lion mark, or CE mark, as these conform to safety standards.*

- *Take care if you buy toys from car boot sales, market stalls or secondhand toys as these may not conform to safety standards and could be dangerous.*

- *Take safety measures such as 'Not suitable for a child under 36 months' seriously (0–3 sign). This sign warns that a toy may be unsuitable for a child under three because of small parts.*

- *Check that the toy has no sharp edges that could hurt your child, or small parts that your child could put in his or her mouth and choke on.*

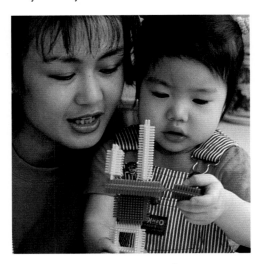

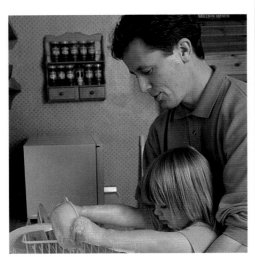

41

'I'd play with them all day if I could. I tell you, it's much more fun than doing the housework.'

'There are things I've got to do. She's forever asking me to play and I'm forever saying "In a minute, in a minute".'

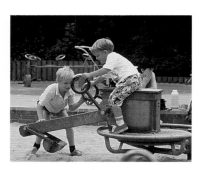

'I don't know that we play all that much. We do a lot of things together, but it's often the shopping and hanging out the washing and that sort of thing. It may not be play, but we have a good time.'

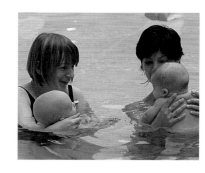

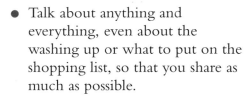

- Talk about anything and everything, even about the washing up or what to put on the shopping list, so that you share as much as possible.

- Find a place and time when your child can learn how to use his or her body by running, jumping and climbing. This is especially important if you don't have much room at home.

- Find other people who can spend time with your child at those times when you really do need to attend to something else.

TOYS FOR CHILDREN WITH SPECIAL NEEDS

Toys for children with special needs should match his or her mental age and ability. They should be brightly coloured and offer sound and action. If a toy made for a younger child is used by an older child, the strength of the toy should be taken into account.

Children who have a visual impairment will need toys with different textures to explore with their hands and mouth. A child who has a hearing impairment will need toys to stimulate language.

MAKING TIME

Some things do have to happen at certain times, and your child does slowly have to learn about that. But when you're with your child try not to work to a strict timetable. Your

child is unlikely to fit in with it and then you'll both get frustrated. A lot of things can be pushed around to suit the mood of you and your child. There's no rule that says the washing-up has to be done before you go to the playground, especially if the sun's shining and your child's bursting with energy.

KEEP YOUR CHILD FIT

Children want to use their bodies to practice until they learn how to crawl, walk, run, jump and climb. The more opportunity you can give them, the happier they'll be, and you'll probably find that they sleep better and are more cheerful and easy going when they've had the opportunity to run off some energy. At the same time you'll be helping their muscle development and general fitness and, if they start to see outdoor activities and sports as a part of their lives, you'll be laying down the habits that will keep them fitter as adults. Make time for your children to exercise.

- Allow your baby to lie and kick his or her legs.

- Make your floor a safe place for a crawler to move around.

- Make time for your toddler to walk with you rather than using the buggy.

- Take toddlers and young children to the park to try climbing and swinging or just so that they have a safe space to run.

- Find out what's on for parents and babies at the local leisure centre.

- Take your baby swimming. There is no need to wait until your child has had his or her immunisations.

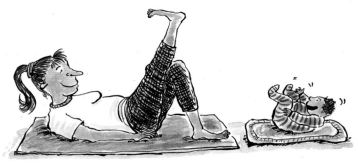

IDEAS FOR PLAY

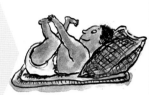
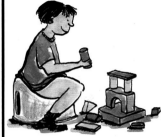
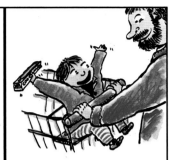

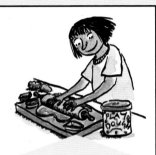
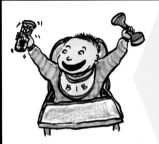

Rattles (from 4 months). Use washed-out plastic screw-top bottles with lentils or dried beans inside. Glue the top securely so it won't come off. Some dried beans are poisonous and small objects can be dangerous for young children.

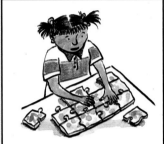

Play dough (from about 18 months). Put 1 cup of water, 1 cup of plain flour, 2 tbsp of cream of tartar, ½ cup of salt, 1 tbsp of cooking oil, and some food colouring or powder paint in a pan. Stir over a medium heat until this makes a dough. Cool. Store in a plastic box in the fridge.

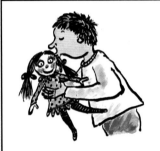
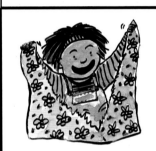

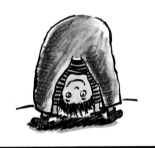
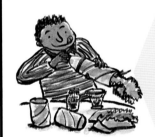

Junk modelling (30 months). Collect all sorts of cardboard boxes, cartons, yoghurt pots, milk bottle tops – anything – and some children's glue, strong enough to glue cardboard, but not to mark clothes. The sort with a brush is easiest to use.

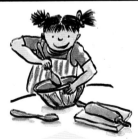
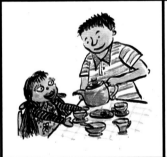
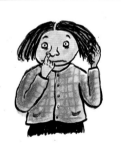
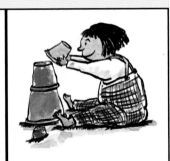

Pretend cooking (from 18 months). Use a bowl, spoons for measuring out and mixing small quantities of 'real' ingredients (flour, lentils, rice, sugar, custard powder) and put out in egg cups or bowls. Use water to mix.

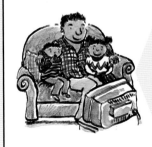

Television gives your child a lot of entertainment, and you a bit of peace. It gives you more peace if it's not on all the time. Make sure you know what your child's watching. And watch with your child when you can so you can talk about what you see.

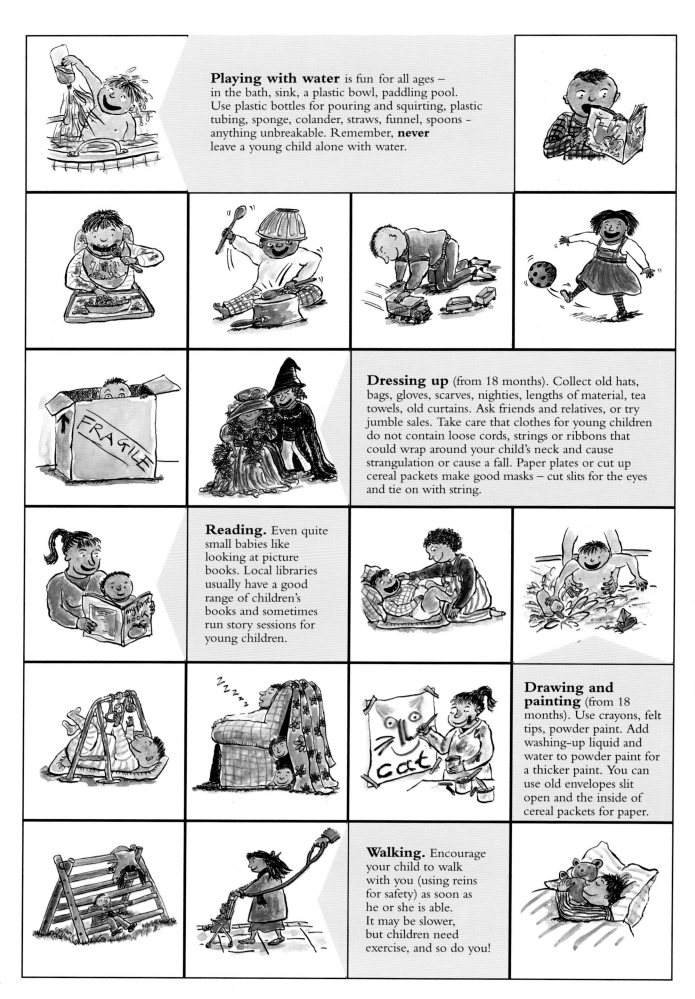

Playing with water is fun for all ages –
in the bath, sink, a plastic bowl, paddling pool.
Use plastic bottles for pouring and squirting, plastic
tubing, sponge, colander, straws, funnel, spoons -
anything unbreakable. Remember, **never**
leave a young child alone with water.

Dressing up (from 18 months). Collect old hats,
bags, gloves, scarves, nighties, lengths of material, tea
towels, old curtains. Ask friends and relatives, or try
jumble sales. Take care that clothes for young children
do not contain loose cords, strings or ribbons that
could wrap around your child's neck and cause
strangulation or cause a fall. Paper plates or cut up
cereal packets make good masks – cut slits for the eyes
and tie on with string.

Reading. Even quite
small babies like
looking at picture
books. Local libraries
usually have a good
range of children's
books and sometimes
run story sessions for
young children.

**Drawing and
painting** (from 18
months). Use crayons, felt
tips, powder paint. Add
washing-up liquid and
water to powder paint for
a thicker paint. You can
use old envelopes slit
open and the inside of
cereal packets for paper.

Walking. Encourage
your child to walk
with you (using reins
for safety) as soon as
he or she is able.
It may be slower,
but children need
exercise, and so do you!

HOW TO MAKE SURE YOUR CHILD LEARNS WHAT YOU WANT HIM OR HER TO LEARN

When children play they're learning what they want. Often these will also be the things you want them to learn, but for some things they may need extra encouragement, like using the potty (see page 51), washing or dressing themselves, learning what not to touch, and where it's not safe to run. It's worth thinking about how you do it.

- **Wait until you think your child is ready.** Forcing something too soon usually ends in failure. You get cross and upset, your child gets cross and upset, and the whole thing becomes impossible. If it doesn't work out, leave it for a few weeks and try again.

- **Try not to make it seem too important.** Your child may learn to eat with a spoon because it's fun, but still want to be fed when he or she is tired, or may enjoy the first few times on the potty because you're so pleased, and then get bored with the idea. In time he or she will see that it is worthwhile learning to be more grown-up and independent.

- **Keep it safe.** If your child is under three years old he or she can't really understand why not to touch your stereo or pull leaves off your pot plants, so keep things you don't want touched well out of the way and you'll both be less frustrated. Time enough to learn about not touching when your child can understand why.

- **Be encouraging.** Your happiness is your child's best reward for good behaviour. If you give your child a big smile, a cuddle or praise when he or she does something right your child is much more likely to try doing it again. Giving your child attention and praise for doing something right works much better than telling him or her off for doing something wrong.

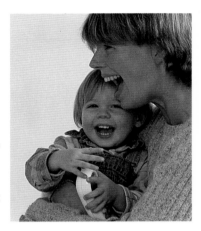

- **Don't ask for perfection** or for instant success. It's safest to expect everything to take much longer than you'd hoped.

- **Set an example.** Whatever it may look like, your child does want to be like you and do what you do. So seeing you wash in the bath, brush your teeth or use the toilet does help.

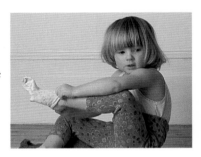

- **Avoid fuss and confrontation.** Once something gets blown up, it can take longer and be much more difficult for everybody to calm down.

- **Be firm.** Children need you to decide some things for them, and need you to stick to your decisions. They need some firm guidelines. So try not to waver. You might start something like potty training, decide your child isn't ready, and give up for a while. That's fine. But a child who is in nappies one day, out the next and back in them the next, is bound to get confused.

- **Be consistent.** For the same reason, it's important that everybody involved in looking after your child is teaching more or less the same things in more or less the same way. If you and your

45

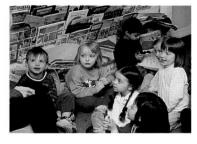

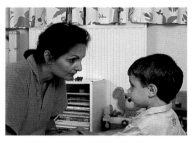

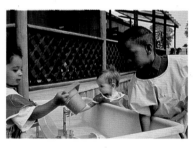

'At playgroup he could run about and make a mess. At home there was just no room. He was happier and I was happier.'

'I would worry about mine being looked after by someone else in case they didn't want to know me.'

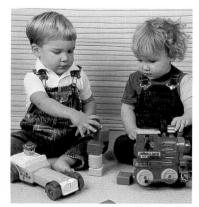

partner, or you and your childminder, do things very differently, your child won't learn so easily and may well play you off against each other.

● **Do what's right for your child, for you and for the way you live.** It doesn't matter what the child next door can or can't do. Don't compete and don't ask your child to compete.

No parent is perfect, and some children seem to find these lessons particularly difficult to learn. See pages 58-64 for dealing with difficult behaviour.

MAKING FRIENDS

Learning how to make friends is one of the most important things your child will do. If your child learns early how to get on well with others he or she will get off to a better start at school, and a happy child learns better than a child who's anxious and afraid of others.

It's never too soon to start, especially if yours is an only child. Even babies and small children like other children's company, although at first they play alongside each other rather than with each other. Ask your health visitor if there's a new parents group meeting in your area. Getting together with other parents can be good for you too (see **Loneliness** on page 122).

As your child starts to crawl and walk you could try a parent and toddler group or a 'one o'clock club'. These can be great for energetic 18 months to three-year-olds, and give you a bit of relaxation and company.

Ask other mothers or your health visitor about groups in your area. Or look on the clinic notice board, or in the newsagent's or toy shop windows. Your local library may also

have information, and may itself run story sessions for pre-school children.

To begin with, your baby or toddler will want you, or another trusted adult, nearby for safety. By the time your child is three, he or she will be ready to spend time without a parent or childminder to run to.

Playgroups, nursery schools or nursery classes all have a lot to offer – more organised play of different kinds, the chance to be with other children and make friends, probably space to run around in.

Find out what's available in your area well in advance as there may be waiting lists. It may be worth putting your child's name down on several lists.

PLAYGROUPS

Playgroups can be found in most areas. They vary in what they offer and how they're run. Some are free, others charge a small fee, though the amount varies. Sometimes you'll be able to leave your child, say for a couple of hours once or twice a week, so you can begin to get your child used to being away from you. Sometimes you'll be asked, or might want, to stay and help. Playgroups are often run by parents themselves. To find out about local playgroups:

● Ask your social services department (Social Work Department in Scotland; Health and Social Services Board in Northern Ireland – see box on page 126) for a list of local playgroups.

● Contact the Pre-school Learning Alliance (formerly The Pre-school Playgroups Association) (address on page 133).

● You could join with other parents to start a playgroup yourself. The Pre-school Learning Alliance can help.

NURSERY CLASSES AND NURSERY SCHOOLS

A nursery class is part of an infant school. A nursery school is a separate school. Not every area has nursery schools or classes and in most areas they only provide sessions of about 2½ hours a day. A few will provide a full school day for four-year-olds. To find out what's available ask your education department, your health visitor or other parents. Local authority nursery schools and classes are free.

INFANT SCHOOL

Legally children must start infant school no later than the beginning of the school term following their fifth birthday. Some schools take children earlier, but an early start isn't necessarily better, particularly if your child hasn't first been to a nursery class and had time to get used to being part of a large group.

Although parents are entitled to choose which school their child goes to, every school has a limit on the number of children it can take. So start looking at schools early, and check with the headteacher whether or not the school is likely to take your child. You can get a list of local schools from your education department (see page 125).

WHEN YOU CAN'T BE THERE

CHOOSING CHILDCARE WHILE YOU WORK

If you're returning to work you'll need to consider how your baby or child will be looked after when you're not there – not just the need

for adults, but also for other children as companions.

Although playgroups and nursery classes rarely keep children for long enough to be useful to a working parent, they can still be used alongside other care from childminders or nannies, so they're worth keeping in mind as you consider your options.

All daycare providers (with the exception of nannies who work in your home) should be registered with your local council social services departments (Or in Northern Ireland your local Health and Social Services Board). Many councils provide handbooks for parents listing all the available care options.

For more on returning to work see page 123.

Childminders

A childminder is usually a mother herself and looks after a small number of children in her own home. Anybody paid to look after children under five in this way for more than two hours a day has, by law, to apply to register as a childminder with the local social services department. This doesn't apply to close relatives, but does apply to friends or neighbours. A childminder is usually registered to care for no more than three children under five, including any of her own. Registered childminders are visited by the social services to check that their homes are suitable and that they can give a good standard of care. So, if you go to a childminder you don't know, make sure that she's registered. You can ask to see her certificate.

You should be able to get the names of childminders with vacancies from your social services department. Other working parents will also be able to tell you about

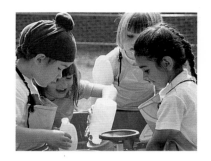

'I wanted him to go to a childminder because I felt if I had to work that was a much more natural setting for him to grow up in ... I don't know, though; maybe a nursery school would have been better where he could have learned to co-operate with people more.'

Before a final agreement is made to place your child with a childminder, ask for a written agreement or contract which safeguards both you and the childminder. It avoids forgetting important things like retainers for holiday periods, extra money for extra time and under what circumstances, payment for any extra expenses, etc. It is easier and makes for a happier relationship if you have a framework.

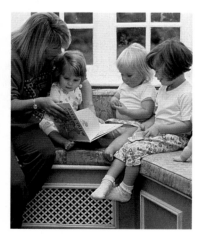

childminders. If you don't already know parents who use childminders, ask your health visitor to put you in touch.

Nannies, mother's helps and au-pairs

Nannies, mother's helps and au-pairs don't have to be registered by the council, which means you don't have the safeguards which the registration of childminders provides. You can contact them through agencies, which will charge you a fee, or through advertisements in your local paper or national magazines. You could try advertising locally yourself.

If you employ a nanny you're responsible for paying her tax and national insurance as well as her wages. You may find that there's another working parent nearby who'd like to share the cost and services of your nanny. **Parents at Work** (see page 133) can provide you with more information on employing a nanny.

Au-pairs are young women or men who come from another country on a one-year basis to learn English. If you invite an au-pair to live in your house he or she should not do more than 35 hours work a week. You provide bed and board and pocket money and access to English lessons in return for help in the home.

Day nurseries

Day nurseries run by local authorities are quite rare. They often have long waiting lists, and only a limited number of places for very young children. Priority is usually given to parents who, for one reason or another, are under a lot of stress and are unable to cope, to parents of children with special needs, and sometimes to working single parents. To get a place at a council nursery, apply to your social services department. Your need will then be assessed by a social worker.

To contact your social services department, look in your phone book under the name of your local authority. (In Scotland the social services department is called the Social Work Department; in Northern Ireland contact your local Health and Social Services Board.)

There may be nurseries in your area run privately or by a voluntary organisation. These nurseries must be registered with a local authority and you can find out about them through your local social services department.

You may be lucky enough to have a nursery or crèche where you work. If one doesn't exist, but there are a number of parents wanting and needing one, it's worth discussing the possibility with your employer. An organisation called Working for Childcare (address on page 133) can give you information.

Sharing/group care

Sharing/group care means getting together with other parents with needs like your own and organising your own childcare. This can work well if at least some of you work part-time. Your health visitor may be able to put you in touch with other parents who work or want to work and need childcare. The Daycare Trust (address on page 133) supplies information about setting up group care. If the group runs for more than two hours a day, and there is any payment involved, it will need to be registered by the local authority. Discuss what this will mean with the under-fives adviser at your local council.

THE COST OF CHILDCARE

The costs of childcare vary and can be very high. You'll have to ask. The cost of a nursery place may depend on your income. It's up to you to agree pay with a childminder, but your social services department may guide you. The National Childminding Association (address on page 133) also gives advice. In some areas, childminding fees are subsidised for low-income or single-parent families.

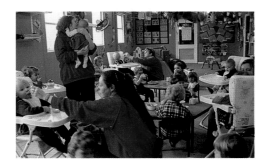

MAKING CHILDCARE WORK

- **First consider your child's needs and what is available.** There are few nursery places for babies and you may prefer leaving a small baby in the care of a single person who you can get to know. A toddler or pre-school child may be happier in a group atmosphere making friends and learning new skills, although a very shy child might prefer, for example, a childminder, but would like to be taken to a playgroup or one o'clock club to meet other children.

- **Your needs are important too.** Will the childcare cover your working hours or will you be looking for someone else to cover the extra time? If the arrangements are too complicated your child may feel anxious and you'll feel very stressed.

- **Before you decide on childcare, visit the childminder or nursery,** talk and ask all the questions on your mind (see the box on page 50 for ideas). Talk about hours, fees, what the fees cover, and what happens during holidays, when there's illness, or an emergency. Write things down as it's easy to forget things.

- **Consider transport arrangements.** How easily can you get there from work and from home?

- **It helps if children can settle in gradually.** If you can, start by leaving your child for a short time and build up. This might mean starting to leave your child before you actually go back to work.

- **Tell your childminder or nursery all about your child,** his or her routine, likes and dislikes, feeding information (particularly if you're still breastfeeding) and so on. When you leave or collect your child, try to make time to talk and find out how things are going.

- **There may be special worries you want to talk about.** If your child has asthma, for example, you'll need to be sure that your childminder doesn't keep pets. You'll also want to know whether the childminder, or any other people in the house, smoke. Or you may need to explain to a white childminder how to do a black child's hair. Perhaps you worry about your child being given certain things to eat. If this is important to you, it's right to talk about it. If childminders don't comply with reasonable requests their registration can be cancelled; consult your local under-fives adviser.

- **Make sure that you and your childminder or nursery workers can agree about issues** such as discipline, potty training and so on.

- **Support and reassure your child in every way you can.** The early weeks are likely to be difficult for both of you. A regular routine, and a handover

'The first day was really terrible. I remember hoping that Andrew's salary would have doubled overnight and that I wouldn't have to go back. But I have to say, now I've got to know the childminder, I enjoy it. And even on the bad days when he's really crying I call the childminder and she says he's settled 10 minutes after I left.'

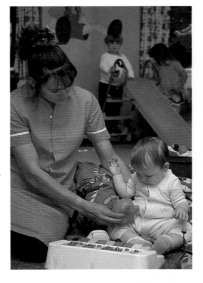

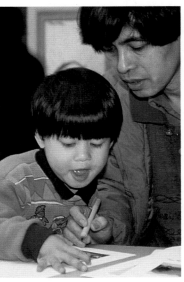

49

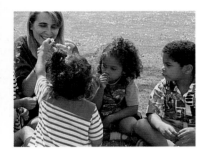

- *How many children are there in a group/ school/class, and how many staff?*

- *How many of the staff are permanent and what are their qualifications?*

- *What would your child's day be like?*

- *What sort of discipline is used?*

- *What facilities are there, such as equipment, space to play outside, space to run around inside when the weather is bad?*

- *Are trips and visits organised?*

- *What teaching is there about different races, cultures and religions?*

- *Are parents expected to help on a regular or occasional basis, perhaps with cooking or outings?*

that's as smooth as possible, both help. Expect crying when you leave, maybe for longer than just the early weeks, but remember the crying usually stops once you've gone. You can ask how long it has gone on. It's best neither to linger long, nor to leave and then go back. Try to keep promises about when you'll return and explain to older children when that will be.

- **Chat with older children about the daily routine,** about the person or people caring for them, about what they've done while away from you. Try to show it's a part of normal life and something to look forward to.

- **It will help you to get into a routine,** and you need to make time with your child part of that routine. A lot of other things will have to go, especially the housework, but not sleep or meals. Share out the work at home with your partner if you can.

- **Children do well in high quality daycare.** So you've no need to feel guilty about not always being there, but if you're worried about the quality of care then it's important to do something about it – talk to child carers, make an unannounced visit during the day and, if necessary, get details of any complaints procedure. Your child depends on you to keep him or her safe, secure and happy.

FINDING A PLAYGROUP, NURSERY OR INFANT SCHOOL

Go to see the group or school
See a few if you have a choice. Talk to the people in charge, look at what's going on, ask questions (see box).

Trust your feelings
If you like the feel of a place and the children seem happy and busy, that's a good sign. You know best the kind of place that will suit your child.

Talk to other parents whose children are at the group or school
Your health visitor may also be able to tell you about other parents' views and experiences.

Talk about ways of settling your child in happily
Staff may suggest ways of helping with this. At a playgroup or nursery school you might, for example, stay with your child at first, and then go away for longer and longer periods. Some children are helped by this sort of gentle start; for others a clean break seems to work best. Some take to change and separation quite easily; others find it hard. Be prepared to give support and reassurance for quite some time if needed.

In some situations, more support and reassurance may be needed. For example, it may be that your child will be one of very few black children at a mainly white school, or one of very few white children. In this situation, talk to the school beforehand about the kind of difficulties that a different colour, culture or language might bring. Find out how the school will handle these, make suggestions yourself if you want to, and explain your child's needs. Talk with your child too, in whatever way seems best.

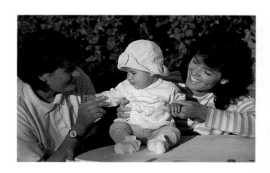

4 Habits and behaviour

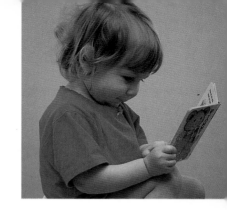

There are some things that our children need to learn just so that we all get along together. The big issues for most parents are that our children should learn to:

- use a toilet
- sleep through the night
- behave reasonably well in public and private.

Sometimes we feel so anxious about these goals that we actually make it harder for our children to achieve them. This chapter helps you to step back a bit and see how you are managing.

POTTIES AND TOILETS

WHAT TO EXPECT

Daytime
Children get bladder and bowel control when they're physically ready for it and want to be dry and clean. The time varies, so it's best not to compare your child with others.

- Most children can control their bowels before their bladders.

- By the age of two, one in two children are dry during the day.

- By the age of three, nine out of ten children are dry most days. Even then all children have the odd accident, especially when they're excited, or upset or absorbed in doing something.

Night-time
Learning to stay dry throughout the night usually takes a child a little longer than staying dry during the day. He or she has to respond to the sensation of having a full bladder while asleep either by waking up and going to the toilet, or holding on until morning. Although most children do learn this between the ages of three and five, it is estimated that:

- A quarter of three-year-olds wet the bed.

- One in six five-year-olds wet the bed.

'It's hard not to push them. You see these other children, you know, younger than yours, and they're all using the potty or the toilet, and there's yours, still in nappies. But they all learn in the end and, looking back, it wasn't that important. At the time I thought it was dreadful because Al was the only child in nappies. But it was only me that minded. Al certainly didn't care, so what does it matter?'

LEARNING TO USE A POTTY

'My mother-in-law kept telling me that all her three were potty trained by a year. At the time, I didn't know whether to believe her or not. I mean, it didn't really seem possible, but I wasn't sure. Looking back now, I suppose she must have spent a lot of time just putting her children on the potty. They didn't really know what they were doing, but if there was something in the potty, she counted that as potty trained. Well, for a start, I haven't got the time or patience for that. And anyway, it doesn't seem worth it. Just catching what comes isn't the same as potty training.'

When to start

It helps to remember that you can't and shouldn't try to force your child to use a potty. In time he or she will want to use it. Your child will not want to go to school in nappies any more than you would want him or her to. In the meantime, the best thing you can do is to encourage the behaviour you want.

Many parents seem to think about starting potty training around 18 to 24 months, but there's no particular time when success is guaranteed. It's probably easier to start in the summer, when washing dries better and there are fewer clothes, if any, to take off.

Try to work out when your child is ready. Most children go through three stages in developing bladder control.

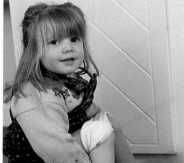

- They become aware of having a wet or dirty nappy.

- They get to know when they are peeing, and may tell you they're doing it!

- They know when they need to pee, and may say so in advance.

You'll probably find that potty training is fastest if your child is at the last stage before you start. If you start earlier, be prepared for a lot of accidents as your child learns.

What to do

- **Leave the potty around where your child can see it and get to know what it's for.** If there are older children around, he or she may see them using it and their example will be a great help. Let your child see you using the toilet and explain what you're doing.

- **If your child regularly opens his or her bowels at the same time each day, take off the nappy and suggest that he or she tries going in the potty.** If your child is the slightest bit upset by the idea just put the nappy back on and leave it a few more weeks before trying again.

- **As soon as you see that your child knows when he or she is going to pee, try the same thing.** If your child slips up, just mop it up and wait for next time. It usually takes a while for your child to get the hang of it and the worst thing you can do is to make your child feel worried about the whole thing.

- **Your child will be delighted when he or she succeeds and a little praise from you will make it better still,** but don't make a big deal of it and don't use sweets as a reward. You may end up causing more problems than you solve.

When the time's right, your child will *want* to use the potty.

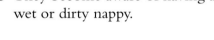

PROBLEMS WITH TOILET TRAINING

Wet children in the day

- **If your child shows no interest in using the potty, don't worry.** Remind yourself that, in the end, your child will want to be dry for him or herself. If your child starts to see the whole business as a battle of wills with you it'll be much harder.

- **Take the pressure off.** This might mean giving up the potty and going back to nappies for a while, or just living a wet life and not letting it get you or your child down. It might help to talk to someone about the best action. What you don't want to do is to confuse your child by stopping and starting too often.

- **Show your child that you're pleased and help your child to be pleased when he or she uses the potty or toilet or manages to stay dry, even for a short time.**
  Be gentle about accidents. You need to explain that it's not what's wanted. But do your best not to show irritation or to nag. Once a child becomes worried, the problem often gets worse.

- **If your child has been dry for a while (night or day) and then starts wetting again, there may be an emotional reason such as a new baby or new house.**
  Be understanding and sympathetic. Your child will almost certainly be upset about the lapse and will not be doing it 'on purpose'.

- **By the time your child starts school he or she is likely to be just as upset by wetting as you are, so do all you can not to be angry.** Your child needs to know you're on his or her side and will help to solve what is now your child's problem more than yours. You can also obtain helpful information from The Enuresis Resource and Information Centre (ERIC) (see page 133 for address).

Bedwetting

Bedwetting up to the age of five is considered normal, and treatment is not usually given. You may, however, find the following measures helpful if your four- or five-year-old wets the bed.

- Try not to get angry or irritated with your child.

- Protect the mattress with a good plastic protective cover.

- Check whether your child is afraid to get up at night – would a night light or potty in the room help?

- **Don't** cut back on fluids as the bladder tends to adjust and holds less. It is better for your child to drink around six or seven cups of fluid during the day so that his or her bladder learns to hold a larger capacity. However, avoid giving fizzy drinks, citrus juices and those with caffeine such as tea, cola and chocolate before your child goes to bed as these can stimulate the kidneys to produce more fluid.

- If your child is constipated, this can also irritate the bladder at night.

Constipation and soiling

Your baby or child is constipated if he or she doesn't empty the bowel properly (some stool stays inside) when going to the toilet . The stool is usually, but not always, hard and difficult to pass. The stools may also look like little pellets.

Most children simply grow out of wetting. If this does not seem to be happening when your child is ready for school, talk to your GP or health visitor about it. You may be referred to a clinic for expert help – not for your sake, but for your child's sake.

If your child continues to be constipated, talk to your health visitor or GP. If it's not sorted out in the end it'll become more of a problem for your child than for you, and he or she may need your help in solving it.

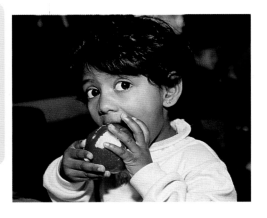

BEDTIME ROUTINE

Establishing a simple routine which your child can identify with and which he or she knows will inevitably lead to going to bed is one of the most important things you can do if your child has a sleep problem.

Another sign of constipation can be if pants are soiled with diarrhoea or very soft stools. This may happen because there is not enough fibre in your child's diet to keep things moving, or it can be something that starts as an emotional problem. Drinking too much milk can also cause constipation.

Once a child is really constipated, even if passing a stool isn't painful, they lose the sensation of wanting to go to the toilet and it needs professional help to sort out.

● If your child becomes constipated, stools can become painful to pass out. The pain means that your child will then hold back even more, become more constipated, have more pain, and so on. It's important to stop this spiral. Ask your health visitor or GP to recommend a suitable laxative. If it doesn't solve the problem quickly, talk to your GP.

● Once the initial problem has been sorted out, it's important to stop it coming back. Make sure your child eats plenty of fibre. Fruit and vegetables, wholemeal bread or chapattis, wholegrain breakfast cereals, baked beans, frozen peas and sweetcorn are good sources of fibre, and children often like them. Also give lots to drink – clear drinks rather than milk. All this will help to prevent constipation.

● If dietary changes aren't helping, consider whether something could be upsetting your child. A young child may be afraid of using the potty. Be reassuring. Let your child be with you when you go to the toilet. And try to be as relaxed as you can be about it.

SLEEPING

In some families, children simply go to bed when they're ready, or at the same time as their parents. Some parents are happy to cuddle their children off to sleep every night. But others want bedtime to be more organised and early enough to give their children a long sleep, and some child-free time for themselves.

Left to themselves most children will get as much sleep as they need. If it doesn't matter to you when that happens, then you're unlikely to regard sleep as a problem.

If, however, your child is staying up late with you but is then regularly woken early perhaps to go to a nursery or childminder, do be sure that he or she is having enough sleep. Your child may need an afternoon nap for longer than a child who regularly goes to sleep at 7.30 pm. Discuss this with your child's carers and make sure that they understand your child's individual needs.

When your child is ready to start school or nursery you may need to think again about late nights. It'll be hard to catch up on sleep in the day and it would be sad if your child was too tired to learn. You may find that bedtime naturally gets earlier as your child adjusts to a more demanding day. If not, you may have to consider being a little more firm about bedtime.

REGULAR BEDTIMES

If you want your baby or toddler to get used to regular bedtimes, be clear, firm and consistent about what you want, and your child will gradually adapt.

- **You stand a better chance of success if he or she is really tired, both mentally and physically.** Try to get outside at least once a day, and not just to give you exercise pushing the buggy. Get your child together with other children – they are good at tiring each other out. Find new activities. A change is often tiring, and something like going swimming can work the odd miracle.

- **Go through the same routine every night,** something like bath, games in the bath, story, quiet time to talk, sleep. Try to make it a time when you give time and attention, but wind down, and don't let the ending go on and on. Make it clear that at a certain point the day must and does come to an end.

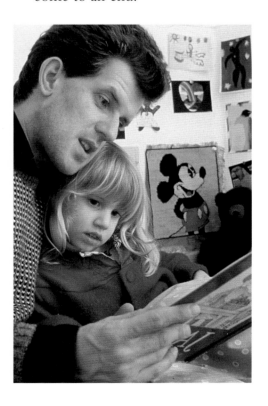

CHILDREN WHO WON'T BE LEFT

If your child won't fall asleep without you then bedtime can become a trying and long drawn-out affair. Try getting your child used to falling asleep alone.

- **One week sit by the bed holding hands. The next week sit further away, and so on.** Don't talk if you can avoid it.

- **Leave a light on.** Perhaps a ceiling or bedside light with a low bulb, or try a dimmer switch. You can also buy glow plugs. They fit into an ordinary socket and give a very low light.

- **Try to get your child to go to sleep with a toy or some kind of comforter instead of you.**

- **Leave the radio or a tape on** (quietly).

- **Leave your child to play for a while if it helps.** Some children settle better if left to play for a while, perhaps in a slightly dimmed light. Other children wind themselves up again this way, and then it's better to take toys out of the room, perhaps leaving one favourite quiet toy and a book.

- **If your child cries or makes a fuss when you leave the room, wait ten minutes, go back, resettle your child the same way as usual, and go away again.** Repeat this as often as you need or can bear, but be firm. You're saying 'I'm still here. I love you, but it's time for sleep.'

- **The important thing is not to give in.** If you've not been firm about bedtimes in the past then your child will expect you to let him or her get up. If this time you

GETTING HELP FOR SLEEP PROBLEMS

Most sleep problems can usually be solved by using simple techniques. But patience, consistency and commitment are usually needed if these have gone on for some time. It is important that both parents should agree on a sleep plan and stick to it.

If you've tried the suggestions on these pages and your child's sleeping is still a problem, talk to your GP or health visitor. They may suggest other solutions or suggest that you make an appointment at a sleep clinic if there is one in your area. Sleep clinics are usually run by health visitors who are specially trained in the management of sleep problems and who can give you the help and support you need. Your GP may also prescribe a drug for very short-term use but it is far better to tackle the long-term issue.

In the meantime, if you're desperate, try to find someone else to take over for the odd night, or even have your child to stay. You'll cope better if you can catch up on some sleep yourself.

Make sure your baby over six months is not waking from hunger. If you gave the last solid food around 5–6 pm, try offering some more food such as bread or a breakfast cereal around 7–8 pm, as well as a milk drink.

OTHER SLEEP PROBLEMS

Nightmares

Most children have nightmares at some stage. They often begin between the ages of 18 months and three years. Nightmares are not usually a sign of emotional disturbance but may occur if your child is anxious about something or has been frightened by a television programme or story.

After a nightmare your child will need comforting and reassuring. If your child has a lot of nightmares and you cannot find the cause, talk to your GP or health visitor.

Night terrors

These can begin under the age of one, but are most common in three-to four-year-olds. They usually start with your child giving a scream or thrashing about while still asleep. He or she may sit up and talk or look terrified while still sleeping.

Night terrors normally have no importance, and your child will eventually grow out of them. Don't wake your child during a terror but, if they happen at the same time each night, try to break the pattern by gently waking your child up about 15 minutes beforehand. Keep your child awake for a few minutes before letting him or her go back to sleep. He or she will not remember anything in the morning.

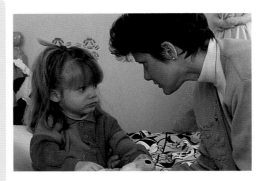

really intend to put a stop to late bedtimes then you must be clear. Give yourself time, try to be as relaxed about it as you can be, and make sure that your partner, or any other adults in the house, will support you.

WAKING IN THE NIGHT

Up to half of all children under five go through periods of night waking. Some will just go back to sleep on their own, others want company. The problem is not so much your child's waking, as your lack of sleep. There are two ways of coping.

Sleep with your child

Some parents like doing this anyway. If you have two children sharing one bedroom, and one is likely to wake the other, it can be the only answer. You may worry that it'll become a habit, and it's true that it may. But if it's a way of getting some sleep, that may be all that matters. It's possible to move some children back to their own beds once they've fallen asleep again and you may be able to teach your child to sleep alone when he or she is old enough to understand what you want.

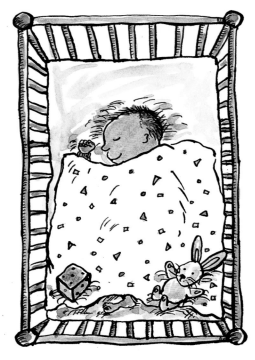

Teach your child to fall back to sleep alone

- **First make sure that your child isn't waking from fear or bad dreams.** Try talking about it. Try and find the reasons – shadows, something seen on television, some family upset – and sort them out if you can. Children don't normally wake from bad dreams much before they are two – and-a-half to three years old.

- **If the reason isn't fear, then try to be firm and fairly brief.** Don't take your child out of the room. Don't start long conversations, stories or games. Try to show that night-time is for sleeping, not company.

- **Make sure your child knows how to fall asleep without you.** If you cuddle or feed him or her to sleep every evening, your child may be unable to get to sleep any other way. Look at the suggestions on page 55 and start by teaching your child to fall asleep alone.

A NEW BABY IN THE FAMILY

Coping with two children is very different from coping with one and it can be tough at first, especially if your first child isn't very old. So far as the baby goes, you've got more experience and probably more confidence, which helps. But the work more than doubles, and dividing your time and attention can be a strain.

It's not unusual for the birth of a second baby to alter your feelings towards your first child. It would be strange if it didn't. At first you may feel that you're somehow not loving your first one as much or enough.

Some parents say they feel very protective towards the baby and 'go off' the older one for a while. It simply takes time to adjust to being a bigger family and loving more than one child.

Your older child, no matter what his or her age, has to adjust too. You can probably help with this, and that will help you.

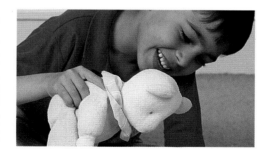

- **Try to keep on as many of the old routines and activities as you can,** like going to play group, going to visit friends, telling a bedtime story. This may not be easy in the early weeks, but it gives reassurance.

- **Don't expect your older child to be pleased with the baby or to feel the way you do.** It's lovely if the pleasure is shared, but best not to expect it.

- **Do expect an older child to be more demanding and to want more and need more of you.** Someone like a grandparent can often help by giving the older one time. But try to give some special attention yourself, and have some time alone together, so your older child doesn't feel pushed out.

- **Older children don't always find babies very loveable, but they often find them interesting.** You may be able to encourage this. There's a lot you can say and explain about babies, and children like to be given facts. Talk about what your older one was like and did as a baby. Get out the old toys and photos. And try to make looking after and playing with the baby a good game, without expecting too much.

- **Feeds are often difficult.** An older child may well feel left out and jealous. Find something for him or her to do, or make feeds a time for a story or a chat.

- **Be prepared for your older child to go back to baby behaviour for a time** – wanting a bottle, wetting pants, wanting to be carried. It's hard, but don't always refuse requests, and try not to get angry.

- **There'll be jealousy and resentment,** shown one way or another, sooner or later. You can only do so much. If you and your partner, or you and a grandparent or friend, can sometimes give each other time alone with each child, you won't feel so constantly pulled in different directions.

'When you've got the one, you don't know how easy it is. Once you've got the two of them, it's much more than twice the work. At the beginning when the second's only a baby still, that's the most difficult time of all.'

'When I only had one, if he had a tantrum, I found I could ignore it and stay fairly calm. Now, with the two of them, if I try to ignore anything, it turns into a full-scale war.'

DEALING WITH DIFFICULT BEHAVIOUR

'I feel split in two. They pull me in different directions the whole time and it's almost impossible to do right by both of them. What's right for the baby is wrong for my older one, and the same the other way round. I love them both, but there doesn't seem any way of showing them that, or of being fair.'

'You get a lot of advice about how to handle your children and I think, because a lot of the time you feel very unsure of yourself, you get to think there's a 'right' way. When you read something, or get a bit of advice, or see somebody handling their child a certain way, you forget to stop and think, you know, 'Is that me?''

'The thing is that what you have to ask of them isn't always what you'd want to ask. It's how things are. My husband works nights and he has to sleep mornings. There's no way round that. If the children are noisy, he can't sleep.'

People have very different ideas about good and bad behaviour. What's bad behaviour to you may be accepted as normal by other parents, and vice versa. Sometimes it's a matter of a particular family's rules. Sometimes it's more to do with circumstances. It's much harder to put up with mess if you haven't got much space, or with noise if the walls are thin.

People react to their children's behaviour very differently. Some are tougher than others, some are more patient than others, and so on. It's not just a matter of how you decide to be. It's also how you *are* as a person.

It's best to set your own rules to fit the way you live and the way you are. And it's best to deal with your child's behaviour your way. But for all parents there will be times when your child's behaviour gets you down or really worries you. There are times when nothing you do seems to work. What do you do then?

UNDERSTANDING DIFFICULT BEHAVIOUR

Try to step back and do some thinking.

Is it really a problem?
In other words, is your child's behaviour a problem that you feel you must do something about? Or might it be better just to live with it for a while? Sometimes it's trying to do something about a certain sort of behaviour that changes it from something that's irritating for you into a real problem for your child. But if a problem is causing you and your child distress, or upsetting

family life, then you do need to do something about it.

It's also worth asking yourself whether your child's behaviour is a problem in your eyes, or only in other people's. Sometimes some kind of behaviour that you can happily ignore, or at any rate aren't worried about, is turned into a problem by other people's comments.

Is there a reason for your child's difficult behaviour?
There usually is, and it's worth trying to work it out before you do anything. Here are just some of the possible reasons for difficult behaviour.

- Any change in a child's life, like the birth of a new baby, moving house, a change of childminder, starting playgroup, or even a much smaller change, can be a big event. Sometimes children show the stress they're feeling by being difficult.

- If you're upset or there are problems in your family your children are likely to pick that up. They may then become difficult at just the time when you feel least able to cope. If a problem is more yours than your children's, don't blame yourself for that. But try not to blame your children either.

- You'll know your child's character and may be able to see that a certain sort of behaviour fits that character. For example, some children react to stress by being loud and noisy and wanting extra attention; others by withdrawing and hiding away.

- Sometimes your child may be reacting in a particular way because of the way you've handled a problem in the past. For example, you may have given your child sweets to keep him or her quiet at the shops, so now your child screams for sweets every time you go there.

- Could you accidentally be encouraging the behaviour you most dislike? If a tantrum brings attention (even angry attention) or night-time waking means company and a cuddle, then maybe your child has a good reason for behaving that way. You may need to try to give more attention at other times, and less attention to the problem.

- Think about the times when the bad behaviour happens. Is it, for example, when your child is tired, hungry, over-excited, frustrated or bored?

CHANGING YOUR CHILD'S BEHAVIOUR

Do what feels right
For your child, for you and for the family. If you do anything you don't believe in or anything you feel isn't right, it's far less likely to work. Children usually know when you don't really mean something.

Don't give up too quickly
Once you've decided to do something, give it a fair trial. Very few solutions work overnight. It's easier to stick at something if you've someone to support you. Get help from your partner, a friend, another parent, your health visitor or GP. At the very least, it's good to have someone to talk to about progress or lack of it.

Try to be consistent
Children need to know where they stand. If you react to your child's behaviour in one way one day and a different way the next, it's confusing. It's also important that everyone close to your child deals with the problem in the same way.

Try not to overreact
This is very hard. When your child does something annoying not just once, but time after time, your own feelings of anger or frustration are bound to build up. But if you become very tense and wound up over a problem, you can end up taking your feelings out on your child. The whole situation can get out of control. You don't have to hide the way you feel. It would be inhuman not to show irritation and anger sometimes. But, hard as it is, try to keep a sense of proportion.

'Your children's behaviour takes over your life. I just felt that I changed totally when I had a second child. I felt my patience had gone completely. If I saw parents shouting in the street I used to think that was a terrible thing. When I had one, I could reason with her and we'd sort it out. When I had two, one only had to do something the slightest bit wrong and I would fly off the handle.'

If you can think about your child's behaviour a bit and begin to understand it, you're more likely to find a right answer. And even if you can't find an answer, you'll probably cope better.

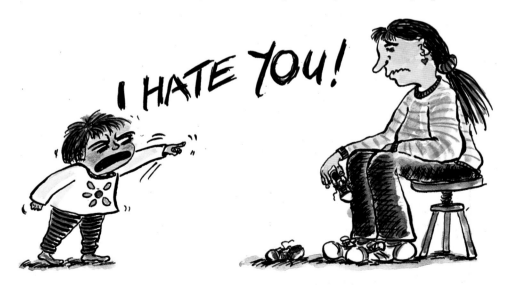

'You think, if I handle this right, they'll learn, it'll get better. But you know sometimes it's just that you have to let time go by. Everything I wanted to happen happened in the end. Sometimes you can try too hard with them.'

'Sometimes I will smack her because she's done something really bad or really dangerous. But other times I know I want to smack her just because of the way I'm feeling, and after, I'll feel bad about it. When it's like that, I just walk away. If John's at home, I'll ask him to take over. And if I'm on my own, I just go into another room and count to ten.'

'It drives me mad. He's plenty old enough to use the toilet, but he won't have anything but the potty, and I'm running around all day emptying it. I had to leave him for a morning with my sister. So I took the potty and told her, you know, I'm sorry, but he won't use the toilet. And when I got back, it turned out he'd gone to the toilet every time, no fuss, nothing said or anything.'

Once you've said what needs to be said and let your feelings out, try to leave it at that. Move on to other things that you can both enjoy or feel good about. And look for other ways of coping with your feelings (see page 61).

Talk

Children don't have to be able to talk back to understand. And understanding might help. So explain why, for example, you want your child to hold your hand while crossing the road, or get into the buggy when it's time to go home.

Be positive about the good things

When a child is being really difficult, it can come to dominate everything. That doesn't help anybody. What can help is to say (or show) when you feel good about something. Make a habit of often letting your child know when he or she is making you happy. You can do that just by giving attention, a smile, or a hug. There doesn't have to be a 'good' reason. Let your child know that you love him or her just for being themselves.

Rewards

Rewards can put pressure on a child, when maybe what's needed is to take the pressure off. If you promise a treat in advance, and your child doesn't manage to 'earn' it, it can cause a lot of disappointment and difficulty. Giving a reward after something has been achieved, rather than promising it beforehand, is less risky. And after all, a hug is a reward.

Smacking

Smacking may stop a child at that moment from doing whatever he or she is doing, but it is unlikely to have a lasting effect. Children learn most by example. If you hit your child you're telling the child that hitting is reasonable behaviour. Children who are treated aggressively by their parents are more likely to be aggressive themselves and to take out their angry feelings on others who are smaller and weaker than they are. Parents do sometimes smack their children, but it is better to teach by example that hitting people is wrong.

WHEN EVERY DAY IS A BAD DAY

No parent 'does it well' all of the time. All parents have bad days, and most go through times when one bad day seems to follow another. Since you can't hand in your notice, or take a week off, you have to find some way of making life work.

When you're tired or in a bad mood, or when your child is tired or in a bad mood, it can be hard to get on together and get through the day. You can end up arguing nonstop. Even the smallest thing can make

you angry. If you go out to work, it's especially disappointing if the short time you've got to spend with your child is spoilt by arguments.

Most children also go through patches of being difficult or awkward over certain things – dressing, or eating, or going to bed at night.

Knowing that it makes you cross or upset probably makes them still more difficult. And you become more and more tense, and less and less able to cope.

REMEMBER

It's all right not to be a 'perfect' parent.

STOP! AND START AGAIN

When you're in a bad patch, a change in routine or a change in the way in which you're dealing with a problem can be all that's needed to stop an endless cycle of difficult behaviour. Here are some ideas.

- **Do things at different times.** An argument that always happens at one time of day may not happen at another. And do the difficult things when your child is least tired or most co-operative. For example, try dressing your child after breakfast rather than before; have lunch earlier, or later. And so on.

- **Find things to do (however ordinary) that your child enjoys, and do them together.** Let your child know that you're happy when he or she is happy. Every time he or she does something that pleases you, make sure you say so. We all prefer praise to blame, and if you give your child lots of opportunities to see you smile the chances are that he or she will learn that a happy mother is more fun than a cross one.

- **Ask yourself whether the thing you're about to tell your child off about really matters.** Sometimes it does, sometimes it doesn't. Having arguments about certain things can get to be a habit.

- **When you lose your temper because you're tired or upset, say you're sorry.** It'll help you both feel better.

- **Don't expect too much.** You may think that sitting still and being quiet is good behaviour. Some children can manage this for a while. Others find it torture because they want to be learning

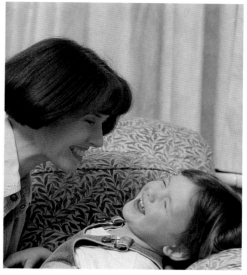

and exploring every waking minute. If your child never keeps still and is 'into' everything, you'll be happier giving him or her as much opportunity as possible to run off steam and explore safely.

- **Don't expect a child under the age of three to understand and remember what they are allowed to do.** Even after the age of three it's hard for a child to remember instructions.

- **Don't expect perfect behaviour.** If you don't expect perfect behaviour then you won't feel so disappointed and angry if you don't get it. After all, if it's all right for you to be a less than perfect parent, then it's all right for your child to be less than perfect too. It's just hard to live with sometimes.

TALK ABOUT IT

It does help to talk and be with other people, especially other parents. It's often true that 'only parents understand'. A lot look very calm and capable from the outside (and you may too), but alone at home most get frustrated and angry at times.

If you don't already know other

'I've just stopped asking myself to be perfect. I've stopped trying so hard. You don't have to be perfect and, if you were, I don't think it would be that good for your child. People have to take me as they find me. That goes for the children, and it goes for people who drop in and find yesterday's washing-up in the sink and a heap of dirty washing on the floor.'

'I think what's so wearing is that it all depends on mood. Not their mood, but mine too. And you have to hide your feelings away so much, and they just let theirs out. If they want to lie down and cry because their favourite T-shirt's in the wash or you won't buy them something at the shops, they just do it. And when they do it in front of other people, that's awful.'

YOU CAN TALK IN CONFIDENCE TO:

- *Parentline 01702 559900 (or see your local phone book)*

- *NSPCC Help Line 0800 800 500*

- *Parents Anonymous 0171 263 8918*

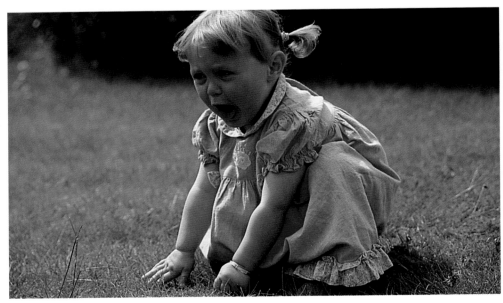

'When it gets too much, I drop everything and get out. I go and see people, find somebody to talk to. I'm a different person when I'm with other people.'

HELP FOR DIFFICULT BEHAVIOUR

You can get help for especially difficult behaviour, so don't feel you have to go on coping alone. Talk to your health visitor or GP, or contact your local child guidance clinic (you can sometimes go without a referral). Sometimes all you need is encouraging support to help you hold on until the problem is over.

Your child can also be referred to a specialist for help. If you've got a special problem, it's right to get special help.

Having a difficult child is an enormous strain. You need help too. See page 61 for more on this.

parents living nearby, look on page 126 for how to find out about local groups. Groups don't suit everybody, but at the very least they're a way of making friends. And a group that is run by parents can often give more than friends who haven't got children the same age. If one doesn't seem right for you it's worth trying a different one.

Sometimes it isn't your child whose mood is a problem. It's you. If you're miserable, trying to be happy for your child's sake may seem impossible. Read Chapter 7 for more about this.

WHEN YOU CAN'T COPE

If every day is a bad day, and you feel that things are getting out of control, *get help*. Talk to your health visitor and/or phone a helpline (see box on page 61). Talking to someone who understands what you're going through may be the first – and biggest – step towards making things better.

Look on pages 133–6 for organisations that provide help and support to new mothers.

TEMPERS AND TANTRUMS

Tantrums may start around 18 months, are common around two years, and are much less common at four. One in five two-year-olds has a temper tantrum at least twice a day. One reason is that around this age children often want to express themselves more than they are able. They feel frustrated and the frustration comes out as a tantrum. Once a child can talk more, tantrums often lessen.

- **Tantrums tend to happen when children are tired or hungry.** Sleep or food might be the answer.

- **If sleep or food isn't the answer, try to work out the reason and tackle that.** It may be frustration. It may be something like jealousy. More time and attention and being extra loving, even when your child is not so loveable, can help.

- Even if you can't be sure why your child has a temper tantrum, try to understand and accept the anger your child is feeling. You probably feel the same way yourself very often. If you think about that, you may be better able to accept your child's feelings.

- **When a tantrum is starting, try to find an instant distraction.** Find something to look at, out of the window for example. Make yourself sound really surprised and interested in it.

- **If your child has a tantrum, try sitting it out.** Don't lose your temper or shout back. Ignore the looks you get from people around you. Stay as calm as you can, try not to get involved, but don't give in. If you've said 'no', don't change your mind and say 'yes' just to end the tantrum. If you do change your mind, your child will think that tantrums pay. For the same reason, don't buy your way out with sweets or treats. If you're at home, you could try walking away into another room.

- **Tantrums often seem to happen in shops.** This can be really embarrassing, and embarrassment makes it extra hard to cope and

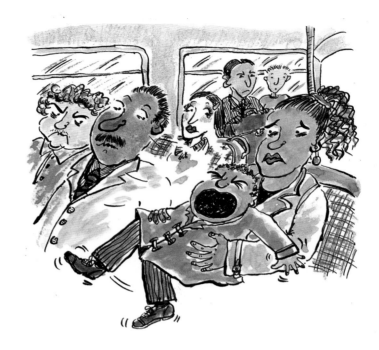

stay calm. Keep shopping trips short. You could start by going out to buy one or two things only, and then build up from there. Once you've managed one quick trip without trouble, you're beginning to make progress.

- **Some parents find it helps to hold their child, quite firmly, until the tantrum passes.** This usually only works when your child is more upset than angry, and when you yourself are feeling calm and able to talk gently and reassuringly.

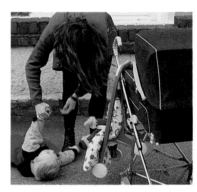

HITTING, BITING, KICKING, FIGHTING

- **Don't hit, bite or kick back.** It makes behaving like that seem all right. You can still make it clear that it hurts.

- **If you're with other children say you'll leave,** or ask others to leave, if the behaviour continues – and do it!

- **Talk.** Children often go through patches of insecurity or upset and let their feelings out by being aggressive – at playgroup, for example. If by talking you can find out what's worrying your child, you may be able to help.

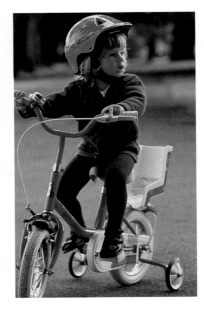

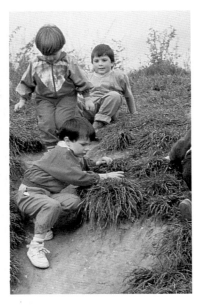

● **Try to show your child how much you love him or her, even though you don't love the way he or she is behaving.** Children who are being aggressive aren't so easy to love. But extra love may be what's needed.

● **Help your child let his or her feelings out some other way.** Find a big space, like a park, and encourage your child to run and to shout. If there's nowhere to run, suggest that he or she shouts and punches a cushion, to get rid of the angry feelings inside. Just letting your child know that you recognise the feelings will make it easier for him or her to express them without hurting anyone else.

OVERACTIVE CHILDREN

There is no doubt that a substantial proportion of children do suffer from hyperactivity or 'Attention Deficit Disorder' as this condition is now called. But quite a lot of children are also extremely active, restless, and difficult to manage *without* suffering from hyperactivity. Or some children may suffer from a *mild* form of hyperactivity. So, the difficulty for parents, and sometimes for health professionals, is deciding what are 'normal' behaviour problems in a child and what are symptoms of Attention Deficit Disorder which require early treatment and management.

Below are some tips on managing an active child. If these, or the other information in this chapter on dealing with difficult behaviour, do not help then talk to your health visitor or GP.

You can also obtain information from the Hyperactive Children's Support Group (see page 133).

● **Keep to a daily routine as much as you can.** Routine can be important if your child is restless or difficult. Routine may also help you stay calmer and stand up better to the strain.

● **Make giving your child time and attention a part of the routine.** In different ways, your child may be demanding your attention most of the day, if not most of the night as well. A lot of the time you'll have to say 'no'. This is easier to say, and may be easier for your child to accept, if there are certain times each day when you do give all your attention to your child.

● **Avoid difficult situations as much as you can** – for example, by keeping shopping trips short. It's often no good even expecting an overactive difficult child to sit still at meals or behave well in a supermarket. And try lowering your expectations. Start by asking your child to be still, or controlled, or to concentrate, for a very short time. Then gradually build up.

● **Try to get out every day to a place where your child can run around and really let go.** Go to a park, or a playground, or whatever safe, open space there is. Find ways of helping your child burn off energy.

● **Try cutting out cola drinks, tea and coffee.** These drinks all contain caffeine. Some children are sensitive to this and it can make them 'jumpy'. So you could try cutting them out and see if it helps.

5 Feeding the family

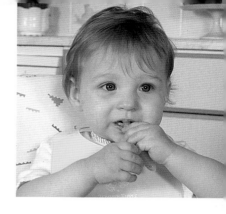

Food is one of life's greatest pleasures and yet it's also a source of worry for most parents. What should children eat? Can I afford to give it to them? Will they eat it? The next few pages will give you some basic guidelines on how to get your baby through the stage of weaning and on to family foods.

STARTING SOLID FOOD

WHEN TO START

For the first four months babies can't properly digest any foods other than breast or formula milk. Some foods, in particular wheat (which is found in several baby cereals), may cause problems well into the future.

Most babies are ready to start solids when they are about four months old. (Babies who were born prematurely will be ready at different times. Ask your GP or health visitor for advice about what is best for your baby.) It's wise to introduce some solids by the time your baby is six months old, as he or she now needs more iron and nutrients than milk alone can provide. Increase solid foods gradually so that between six and twelve months these become the main part of the diet, with breast or formula milk to drink alongside. If weaning is delayed after six months, some babies also have difficulties in eating foods with lumps and will only accept purées.

'With your first baby, you worry about what you give them, and how much, and whether they'll like it But with your second, it's much more like they have to fit in with the rest of the family, and you don't think about it so much. They take what's going, and they do it for themselves really.'

'I think there's a lot of pressure on you to stop the breastfeeding and, you know, get on to something a bit more substantial. People are always sort of pushing you on to the next stage. It's hard to know what's best when people are saying to you "Isn't she weaned yet?" and "Have you tried this, have you tried that?"

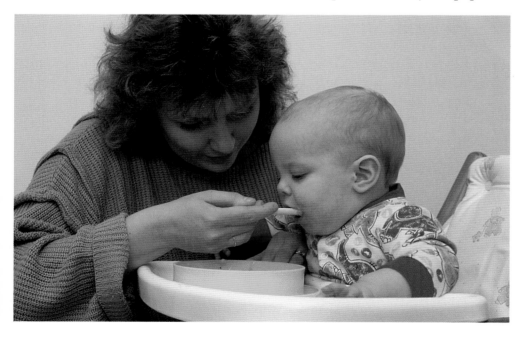

HOW CAN YOU TELL WHEN YOUR BABY IS READY?

Your baby is ready to start solid food if he or she is between four and six months old and

- *seems hungrier than usual*

- *starts to demand feeds more often*

- *starts waking again to be fed, after sleeping through the night.*

If you have any doubts, talk to your health visitor.

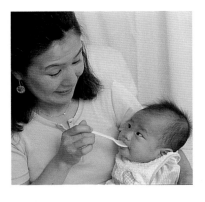

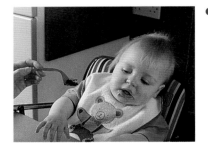

GUIDELINES

All babies are different. Some start solid food earlier, some later. Some take to it quickly, some take longer. Some are choosy, others like anything and everything.

- **Go at your baby's pace.** Until now your baby has only known food that is a liquid and comes from a nipple or a teat. Your baby needs to learn to move solid food from the front of his or her tongue to the back in order to swallow it. What you're doing is teaching your baby to take and enjoy food that has a different taste, a different feel, and comes in a different way. This is bound to take time.

- **In the end, you want your baby to be eating like the rest of the family.** So your baby needs to learn to like a variety of ordinary foods. In any case, variety early on might mean you avoid choosiness later. Your baby also needs to adapt to the family pattern of eating - say, three meals a day with a drink at each and two or three additional snacks - which will take time.

- **From the start, try not to rush and don't 'force feed'.** Most babies know when they've had enough to eat. Don't spend a lot of time persuading your baby to take food. Babies soon learn that refusing food is a good way of getting attention – or of getting a sugary pudding instead of a savoury first course! Of course it's right to give attention, chat and enjoy meals together. But when food is refused, it might be best to call an end to the meal.

- **When your baby shows an interest in feeding him or herself, this is a good sign.** Encourage this by giving your baby one spoon whilst you try to spoon in most of the meal. It will be messy at first so put newspaper on the floor and try not to worry about the mess.

- **Make sure everything you use for feeding your baby is really clean.** Spoon out the amount of food you think your baby will eat and warm this, rather than heating a large amount. You can always heat up more but it's not safe to reheat previously warmed food. Heat food really thoroughly and allow to cool, and don't refreeze warmed food if it isn't used. **Saliva contains factors which can cause food to go off, so throw away any food your baby hasn't eaten.**

- **Commercial baby foods can be useful, but don't let them replace home-made foods altogether.** Use mashed up family food when you can – it will get your baby used to eating what you eat. When you use commercial baby foods, follow the mixing instructions carefully and check the expiry date and that the seals on jars and cans haven't been broken. Look at the labels, first to check if the food is suitable for your baby's age and stage of weaning, and secondly to check for unnecessary added sugars (see page 76-77 for more about sugar).

- **Always use a separate plate and spoon for your baby.**

- **Take care to heat foods safely for your baby.**

STARTING SOLID FOODS

THE FIRST TWO WEEKS OF WEANING

Start with a little smooth vegetable or fruit purée with no added salt or sugar, or cereal (not wheat-based) on the tip of a clean teaspoon or your finger. Just a small teaspoonful is enough at first. Offer it to your baby before or after one of the milk feeds in the day, or in the middle of the feed if that works better. If you heat the food, make sure it's not too hot when you give it. If you use a microwave oven, be sure to stir well (parts of the food may be very hot even though other parts will be cool).

Most babies take time to learn how to take food from a spoon. Be patient and prepared for some spitting and mess. Your baby may at first also cry between mouthfuls. Until now, food has come in one continuous stream. Now there are frustrating pauses.

Don't press the food on your baby. If it really doesn't seem to be wanted, give up. Wait until next time. The main aim at this stage is to get your baby used to the idea of taking food from a spoon and your baby should still be having breast milk or 600 mls (around a pint) of formula milk a day.

Foods you might try
● Vegetable or fruit purées such as potato, carrot, yam, plantain, courgette, cooked apple, banana.

● Thin porridge (made from rice, cornmeal, sago, millet), mixed with formula or breast milk.

● Baby rice and other first baby foods you can buy (use the instructions on the packet to make these up).

Don't yet give
● Wheat-based foods such as wheat flour, breakfast cereals, rusks etc
● nuts and seeds, e.g. sesame (see page 79) ● eggs ● fish and shellfish ● citrus fruits and juices
● follow-on milk ● cow's milk
● milk products, e.g. yoghurts and custards if your family has a history of allergies ● salt ● sugar
● honey ● chillies or strongly spiced food. These foods could upset your baby or trigger an allergy (see **Food allergies** on page 79).

THE NEXT 6 TO 8 WEEKS

Feeds will still be mainly breast or bottle, but now very gradually increase the amount of solid food you give either before, during or after the milk feed. Try to follow your baby's appetite. Give the amount that seems to be wanted.

At the same time, move gradually from solid food at one feed in the day to solid food at two, and then three feeds. You will find that as your baby eats more solid food, his or her milk intake will start to decrease. Once he or she is on three meals a day you can drop one milk feed, but your baby should still be having breast milk or 500–600 ml (about a pint) of formula a day. Full fat cow's milk products can be used in weaning after four months (for example, yoghurt, custard or cheese sauce). Again, try to follow your baby's appetite and go at your baby's pace.

Try to keep cereals for one feed only. Begin to add different foods and different tastes. You'll be able to use lots of the foods you already cook for yourself. Just mash, sieve or purée a small amount (without added salt or sugar) and give it a try.

Using your own family food is cheaper, you know what the

It can be useful to have a few jars or packets of baby food in the cupboard, but don't let them replace home-made foods altogether. Use puréed or mashed up family foods when you can — it's cheaper, you know what the ingredients are, and it will get your baby used to eating what you eat. If you buy baby foods:

● *check they are suitable for your baby's age, e.g. from four or seven months;*
● *check the expiry date;*
● *check the seals on cans and jars haven't been broken;*
● *avoid these foods before 6 months: wheat-based foods which contain gluten, nuts, seeds, eggs, fish citrus fruits and juices — check the label for these;*
● *choose foods which state they do not contain added sugars*
● *baby foods are not allowed to contain salt, but ingredients such as bacon and cheese will contain some;*
● *if your family has asthma, eczema or allergies to foods, talk to your GP or health visitor to see if your baby needs to avoid other foods;*
● *rusks contain wheat (unless 'gluten-free') and sugar;*
● *'baby muesli' may contain nuts and wheat. Check the list of ingredients and avoid these if your baby is under six months. You may also wish to avoid giving nuts to an older baby (see page 79);*
● *'mixed cereals' are likely to contain wheat. Avoid these if your baby is under six months.*

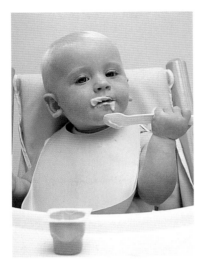

ingredients are (halal meat, for example) and your baby will get used to eating like the rest of the family. Although you should stick to breast or formula milk for your baby's main drink, you can, if you wish, start to use full-fat cow's milk for cooking.

Foods you might now add
● Purées using meat (including liver) ● Poultry ● Split pulses such as lentils ● A wider variety of vegetable and fruit purées ● Full-fat milk products – yoghurt, fromage frais, custard – unless your family has a history of eczema, asthma or other allergies.

Still avoid
● Wheat-based foods (including bread and rusks) ● Eggs ● Citrus fruits ● Nuts and seeds (e.g. sesame) ● Fatty foods ● Chillies and other strong spices ● Fish and shellfish ● Honey (see page 70).

FROM 6 TO 9 MONTHS

You can now move from purées to food that's just mashed or minced. Most babies can start to chew soft lumps from six to seven months even if they have no teeth. Once your baby has grown used to a variety of foods give the solids first and the milk feed second.

From six months, in addition to breast milk or a minimum of 500-600ml (around a pint) of formula or follow-on milk, you can start to add a wider range of foods, including wheat-based foods such as flour, bread and wholewheat breakfast cereals. Try to give at least two to three servings daily of starchy foods such as potatoes, rice, unsweetened breakfast cereals, yams and bread.

As solid food becomes a large part of your baby's diet it is important to offer a range of different foods to provide the vitamins and minerals he or she needs. Every day include two servings of fruit or vegetables and one serving of soft cooked meat, fish, pulses such as lentils (dahl) or well cooked egg.

Dairy products such as full-fat cheese, full-fat plain yoghurt and fromage frais are a good source of calcium, so include these too. Full-fat pasteurised cow's milk can also be used for mixing food such as cereal but not as a drink until 1 year old. It does not have to be boiled.

Finger foods and 'lumps'
Food should now be made a little lumpier to encourage your baby to start to chew. (Start with 'soft lumps'.) Otherwise you may find your baby refuses to eat 'lumpy food' as he or she gets older. Chewing also encourages the development of the speech muscles. Once your baby can hold things, try finger foods such as toast, a crust of bread, bread sticks, a piece of pitta bread or chapatti, a slice of peeled apple or banana, or a raw or cooked carrot or green bean. These provide good chewing practice and will help your baby learn to feed him or herself. **Stay nearby in case of choking.** Avoid sweet biscuits or rusks, so that your baby does not get into the habit of expecting sweet snacks. Even low sugar rusks contain sugar.

Drinks
Keep to your baby's usual milk or water for a drink. If you do use pure fruit juice, dilute it one part juice to 10 parts water and give it with meals in a lidded cup. After six months, tap water need not be boiled.

You can now add
● Citrus fruit ● Well cooked eggs ● Wheat based foods ● Oily fish and shellfish ● Ground nuts and peanut butter if there are no allergies in your family (see page 79).
In other words, you can now give almost any family food provided you make it the right consistency for your baby.

Still avoid
● Nuts and seeds (e.g. sesame seeds) if your child has allergies such as hayfever, eczema or asthma or if there are allergies in the family ● honey.

FROM 9 TO 12 MONTHS

By now your baby will be eating many family foods, although you will still have to chop or mince some foods. It is still important for your baby to have breast milk or around 500–600 mls (around a pint) of formula or follow-on milk a day. In addition, make sure your baby has other dairy products such as full fat plain yoghurt, fromage frais or cheese.

He or she will need three to four servings of starchy foods (bread, potatoes, breakfast cereals, rice, pasta, maize, etc.) a day – you can include one or two wholemeal varieties occasionally if your child is eating well. Don't encourage a sweet tooth by giving biscuits and cakes, and only add sugar if really necessary (for example, to sour stewed fruit).

Still avoid
● Nuts and seeds, e.g. sesame (see page 79), if your child has allergies such as hayfever, eczema or asthma or there are allergies in the family ● honey.

FROM 12 MONTHS ONWARDS

Your baby should be having a good mixed diet by now, with probably three meals and a couple of healthy snacks in between (see box on page 76). You can now transfer your baby from infant formula or follow-on milk to full-fat cow's milk, and should try to make sure he or she has around 350 ml (12 oz) of milk a day to drink. Carry on breastfeeding if you wish.

If your baby is reluctant to drink milk, make sure he or she has at least two servings of yoghurt or cheese or milk-based dishes (such as cheese sauce, custard, rice pudding) a day.

Your baby's diet should contain plenty of starchy foods and a wide range of fruit and vegetables now – four servings of each a day – and one or two servings of meat, fish or eggs. Encourage your baby to eat oily fish such as canned sardines, pilchards, salmon and mackerel and use lean cuts of meat. If your baby has a meat and fish-free diet, give diluted fruit juice with every meal to help absorb iron from foods.

Which foods should I avoid giving?
Some foods are thought to be more likely to upset a baby or cause an allergic reaction than other foods. These include **citrus fruit, nuts, seeds (e.g. sesame), eggs, fish, shellfish and wheat.** So avoid giving any foods which contain these ingredients until your baby is at least six months old. Then you can introduce, one by one, small amounts of citrus fruit, well cooked eggs (cooked until the white and yolk are solid) and wheat products such as flour, bread and pasta, checking to make sure there is no reaction.

If someone in your family has asthma, eczema or other allergies, it is probably best to talk to your GP or health visitor before introducing these foods (see page 79). If someone in your family can't eat foods containing gluten, also talk to your GP before giving any wheat, rye or barley-based foods.

● **Salt** Don't add any **salt** to baby foods, as your baby's kidneys can't cope with it, and it is best not to encourage a liking for salt. When you're cooking for the family leave out the salt, so baby can share the food. (It's better for all of you without the salt anyway.)

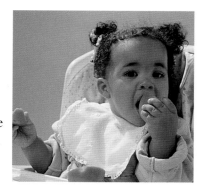
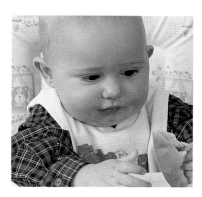
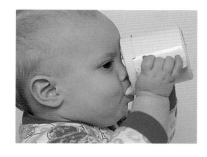
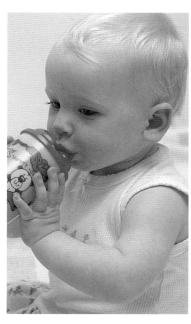

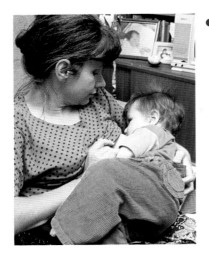

HANDY HINTS FOR
WEANING

- *Allow plenty of time for feeding particularly at first.*

- *Introduce new foods mixed with familiar ones.*

- *Always stay nearby whilst your child is eating.*

- *Try not to get upset if the food is refused – just take the food away and try again later.*

- *Prepare larger quantities of food than you need and freeze small portions of it for later use.*

- *Cover the floor with newspaper and use a bib to catch food spills – weaning is a messy business! Allow plenty of time for feeding particularly at first.*

- **Sugar** Avoid adding **sugar** to any foods or drinks your baby has, as it could encourage a sweet tooth and lead to tooth decay when the teeth first start coming through. (If stewing fruit which is sour, eg rhubarb add as little sugar as possible, or mash in a little banana or a small amount of breast or formula milk.) Encourage your baby to eat savoury foods and if buying baby food use sugar-free varieties.

- **Honey** Also avoid using spoonable or set **honey** even for easing coughs or restlessness until your baby is at least a year old. Not only is honey a sugar, but very occasionally it may contain a type of bacteria. If eaten by a baby under the age of one, these can grow and produce toxins in the baby's intestine. This could result in a potentially serious illness to your baby called 'infant botulism'. After the age of one, the intestine matures and the bacteria are not able to grow.

- **Cow's milk and goat's or sheep's milk** are not suitable as drinks for babies under one year as they do not contain enough iron and other nutrients for proper growth. You can give them after the baby is one year old if they are full fat milk and have been pasteurised or boiled.

- **Soya milk** can also cause allergic reactions, and if a soya-based milk is recommended by a paediatrician or dietitian instead of cow's milk formula, you should use a special infant formula soya milk (see page 72).

- **Nuts and seeds** can provoke a life- threatening reaction in the few people who are allergic to

them. Whole peanuts should *not* be given to children under five years old as they can choke on them. *Avoid* giving nut or seed butters until babies are at least six months old. If there is a family history of allergies (including eczema, asthma and hayfever) avoid giving peanuts and foods containing peanut products until at least 3 years of age (see page 79).

WEANING FROM THE BREAST OR BOTTLE

You can go on breastfeeding your baby alongside giving solid food for as long as you want to. If both you and your baby enjoy it, there's no reason to stop. A bedtime breastfeed can make a good end to the day.

Continuing breastfeeding or using infant formula (or follow-on milk after the first six months) during the first year ensures a good source of nutrients as well as being convenient and cheap.

If you use a bottle or trainer cup don't put anything in it other than formula or breast milk. Comfort sucking on sweetened drinks is the major cause of painful tooth decay in young children. It's a good idea anyway to wean from a bottle by the end of the first year as bottle-sucking can become a habit that is hard to break. There is also an increased incidence of glue ear in babies who suck from bottles.

It's a good idea to teach your baby to use a lidded feeding cup to give milk or water any time after six months. Offer the breast or bottle as well at first, and gradually cut down. Or, if you think this puts your baby off the cup because there's something 'better' coming afterwards, try cutting out the breast or bottle feed at one meal in the day and using the cup instead.

VITAMINS

Parents are sometimes confused about whether or not to give their baby vitamin drops. Your health visitor should be able to advise you. Generally, however, if you are still breastfeeding after your baby is six months old, he or she should have baby vitamin drops containing vitamins A, C and D. If your baby is bottle fed and having more than 500 mls of infant formula or follow-on milk a day, he or she will not need vitamin drops. If he or she is drinking less than this, then it would be sensible to give vitamin drops. These can normally be obtained cheaply from child health clinics, or are free if you qualify (see page 131).

When you stop giving infant formula or follow-on milk (any time after your baby is one year old), it is sensible to give vitamin drops up to the age of five unless you know that your child eats plenty of food containing vitamins A, C and D (see box) and regularly gets out into the sunshine.

Sunshine helps make vitamin D which is important in making strong bones. As little as half an hour playing outdoors is sufficient to meet your child's vitamin D requirement. See page 104 for advice about safety in the sun. Children who wear clothes that cover them right up throughout the year when outdoors, may not get enough vitamin D, so should have vitamin drops until they are five years old.

ANAEMIA

Newborn babies have a store of iron that lasts about six months. Between 6 and 12 months it's important to prevent anaemia which can hold back their development. Babies can get iron from:

- a good mixed diet which includes meat and/or pulses and dark green vegetables;

- infant formula and follow-on milk (which have added iron) as their main drink.

If you are continuing breastfeeding and would prefer a vegetarian diet for your baby, make sure that it contains plenty of foods which are high in vitamin C as this helps the body absorb iron.

Don't give any other vitamin supplements (such as cod liver oil) in addition to vitamin drops. Too much of some vitamins is as harmful as not enough.

'Yes, I want my kids to eat the right sort of things. But wanting is one thing and doing it, or getting them to do it, is something else altogether. Mostly what one will eat the other won't. The only things I know they'll both eat are things like chips and sausages. Family meals almost always mean one of them making a fuss. You can make something for them that takes twice as long as sausages or whatever, and you end up putting it all in the bin.'

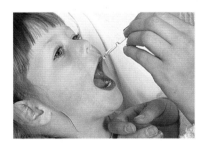

SOURCES OF VITAMIN A	SOURCES OF VITAMIN C	SOURCES OF VITAMIN D
dairy products	*oranges (not suitable for under 6 months) and juice*	*sunshine*
fortified margarine		*fortified margarine*
liver	*strawberries, kiwifruit, blackcurrants, mangoes*	*fortified breakfast cereal*
carrots and dark green vegetables (cabbage / spinach / broccoli)	*broccoli, peppers*	*canned salmon, sardines, tuna*
	peas, cauliflower, cabbage, nectarines, tomatoes	*meat*

DRINKS

MILK

Never give your baby or toddler juice or squash to drink from a bottle, even if you are out with your child. Drinking juice from a bottle continually bathes the teeth in sugar and can cause tooth decay. It can also fill your child up and lessen his or her appetite for food. If you give these drinks only give them from a cup at mealtimes.

- **Breast milk** is the best source of nourishment in the first few months of life. If you breastfeed, try to do so for at least four months, and ideally for a year, especially if your family has a history of allergies, eczema or asthma. You can go on breastfeeding for as long as you want to.

- **Infant formula** based on cow's milk is the only alternative to breastfeeding in the first six months and this can be used up to the time when ordinary cow's milk can be introduced (at one year). Some mothers like to swap to **follow-on milks** after their baby reaches six months, but this is not necessary. Don't give your baby flavoured milk.

- **Soya milk** If your baby is using a **soya-based infant formula** you will need to be particularly careful about his or her teeth once they start coming through. Soya formulae contain sugars which can cause decay, so you should keep drinks of soya formula to mealtimes, and avoid allowing your baby to suck for long periods on a bottle (for example, as a comforter). Try to cut out a bedtime bottle or clean baby's teeth afterwards. When your baby reaches one year, use a cup not a bottle because it cuts down the amount of time teeth are in contact with the sugars in the milk. If you are weaning your baby on to a vegan (strict vegetarian diet), you should continue using the soya-based formula until the age of two as it is a good source of many important nutrients.

- **Full-fat cow's milk** can be used in cooking once your baby has started weaning or from 6 months if your family has a history of eczema, asthma or other allergies. But it is not suitable for a main drink for your baby until he or she is one-year- old as it doesn't contain sufficient iron and other nutrients for your baby's needs. For convenience, lower-fat milk can be used in cooking after the age of one. Semi-skimmed milk is not suitable as a main drink for children under two, and **skimmed milk** is not suitable for children under five.

OTHER DRINKS

It's a good idea to start using a lidded feeding cup for milk or water from the age of six months, and try to wean your baby off bottles by the time he or she is one. Do this gradually by offering the breast or bottle as well at first, or just giving a cup at one mealtime a day.

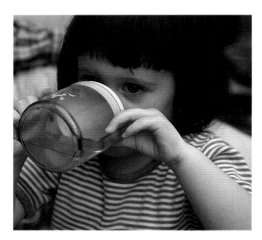

- **Milk and cooled boiled water** are the best drinks for your baby. Other drinks can fill babies and toddlers up leaving them with little appetite for more valuable foods and milk at mealtimes.

- **Citrus fruit juices** (e.g. orange, grapefruit) are a good source of vitamin C but also contain naturally present sugars which can cause tooth decay. However, the vitamin C they contain will help any iron in the meal to be readily absorbed. Your health visitor may therefore advise that you give fruit juice with your child's meal to help iron absorption, especially if you are bringing your baby up as a vegetarian or are breastfeeding. Give very dilute (one part pure fruit juice to 10 parts water) from a cup at meal times once your baby has reached six months. Toddlers can have juice diluted one part juice to 5 parts water.

- **Squashes and other drinks such as non-diet fizzy drinks, flavoured milk, and juice drinks** contain sugars, and even if diluted can cause tooth decay. Filling up on too much squash can also result in poor appetite, poor weight gain and, in toddlers, loose stools . If you want to use them, keep them for mealtimes and offer water and milk in between. *Never give them as a bedtime drink or put in a bottle for your baby to hold, and try to keep drinking times short.*

- **Diet drinks,** whether squashes or fizzy drinks, are not intended for babies and toddlers. They contain artificial sweeteners which may be more tooth friendly than other squashes but can still encourage a sweet tooth. Frequent consumption of artificially sweetened drinks by children could result in excessive intakes of saccharin. They can also give toddlers diarrhoea. Dilute these by at least 10 parts water to one part sweetened drink.

- **Fizzy drinks** – *don't* give toddlers these. They are acidic and can damage tooth enamel.

- **Bottled 'natural mineral water'** is *not* safe for babies to use as it can contain very high levels of some minerals, such as salt. Carbonated (that is fizzy) water is also unsuitable for babies. If for any reason you need to use mineral water for your baby (for instance when travelling abroad) check what type to use with your health visitor.

- **'Baby' and herbal drinks** may contain sugars and their use is *not* recommended.

- **Goat's and sheep's milk** don't contain enough iron and some important vitamins to make them suitable for children under one year. Provided they are boiled or pasteurised full fat varities can be used once a baby is one year old.

- **Tea and coffee are not suitable drinks for babies or young children.** They reduce iron absorption when taken with meals, and if sugar is added, may contribute to tooth decay.

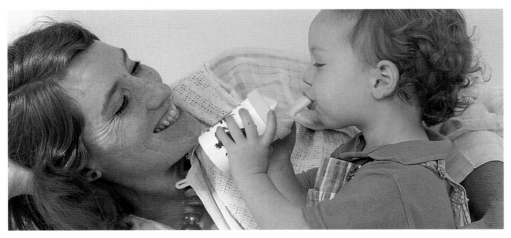

FAMILY FOOD

Children under two need the extra fat and vitamins in full-fat dairy products, so don't give semi-skimmed milk, diet fromage frais, diet yoghurts, reduced fat spreads or cheeses. Skimmed milk is not suitable for children under the age of five. After the age of two, low-fat milk can be used in family cooking for convenience.

'It's difficult to give them healthy food because of the money. But some of the stuff that's not healthy costs most of all – like sweets. And there are things you can do – like beans and lentils and things are cheap and you can store them. And I slice up fruit and share it between the kids and it goes further.'

'I do feel, you know, I wish she'd eat that. But I'm resigned to it. Because even getting her to try things is hard. So I just serve up the same old things, and it's a fairly good mix, so why worry? I mean, she does eat different sorts of food. She eats baked beans, she loves bread, she'll drink milk. Potatoes and cheese always go down OK. She has orange juice and apples, bananas sometimes. There's nothing wrong with that.'

For most people the move towards a healthy, balanced diet means eating more bread, breakfast cereals, potatoes, pasta and rice and more fruits and vegetables. The plate below shows the types of foods and proportions you need to eat them in to have a well-balanced, healthy diet.

This is the type of diet adults and children over the age of five should be eating. Children aged between two and five will be eating a diet which is higher in fat and lower in fibre that this, but by five should be eating a similar diet to adults.

WHAT SHOULD TODDLERS EAT?

We all need energy (calories) and nutrients (protein, carbohydrate, fat, minerals and vitamins) to grow, for activity, and for the body to work properly and repair itself. Babies and children under the age of two have small tummies and can't eat large amounts of food all in one go, so they need small meals with healthy snacks in between. Foods which are a concentrated source of energy and nutrients such as milk, dairy products, meat, oily fish and eggs should be an important part of their diet, with plenty of starchy foods and fruit and vegetables besides.

FAT AND FIBRE

Some people wrongly think that small children need a low-fat diet, just like adults. Children under the age of two need fat in their diet to provide energy, and some vitamins are only found in fat. It is therefore much more important to make sure that they eat a variety of foods and get enough calories than to worry about fat. Between the ages of two and five their diet can gradually change to be more like that of an adult that is lower in fat, especially saturated fat.

It is also a mistake to give babies and toddlers a high fibre diet as it is quite bulky and can stop important minerals like calcium and iron from being absorbed. Higher fibre foods such as wholemeal bread, pasta and brown rice can be gradually introduced, so that by the time children are five they are used to a healthy adult diet.

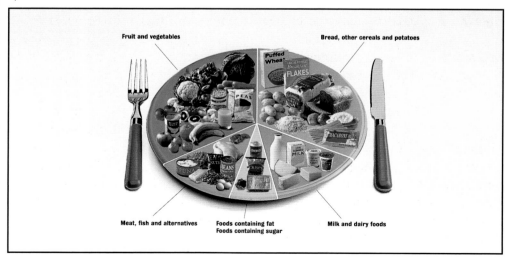

Fruit and vegetables

Bread, other cereals and potatoes

Meat, fish and alternatives

Foods containing fat
Foods containing sugar

Milk and dairy foods

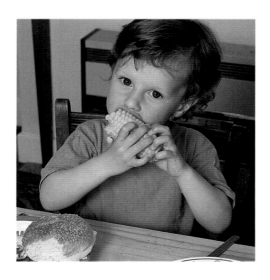

Your toddler's diet

Like the rest of the family, your toddler needs to eat a variety of foods from four groups of food. By doing this your child will almost certainly get all the nutrients he or she needs:

- **Milk and dairy foods** – milk, cheese, yoghurt, fromage frais.

- **Meat, fish and alternatives** – meat, fish, poultry, eggs, beans, lentils, etc.

- **Bread, other cereals and potatoes** – bread, rice, pasta, maize, potatoes, breakfast cereals etc.

- **Fruits and vegetables** – all types of fruits and vegetables.

The fifth group of foods – **foods containing fat and foods containing sugar** – are enjoyed by children and adults alike, but don't contain many nutrients, so limit how often your toddler eats biscuits, cakes, chocolate, puddings, sweets, ice cream and fat spreads.

Milk and dairy foods

Milk and dairy foods such as cheese, yoghurt and fromage frais contain protein, vitamins and also zinc, and are an excellent source of calcium which is needed for bones and teeth.

Offer your child milk (breast, formula or follow-on up to one year) instead of juices to drink. If your child is reluctant to drink milk, make sure he or she has plenty of other dairy foods.

Milk and dairy products are also a good source of vitamin A, which helps the body resist infection and is needed for healthy skin and eyes.

Meat, fish and alternatives

This group of foods contains protein and important minerals such as iron and zinc. It includes meat such as beef, pork and lamb, chicken and turkey, liver, kidney, sausages, burgers and meat pies; fish, whether frozen, canned or fresh or fish fingers; eggs, beans and lentils, textured vegetable protein and other meat alternatives (tofu, quorn, etc.); and nuts. Some of these foods are unsuitable for children under six months - see page 67.

Try to give meat, fish, eggs or poultry at one meal a day, or beans, lentils, tofu, etc. at two meals a day. It doesn't have to be expensive to be nutritious. Baked beans or sardines on toast are both nutritious and cheap, and an egg is quickly cooked for breakfast or tea.

Meat and fish help to increase the amount of iron absorbed from other foods eaten at the same meal, so try to give some every day. They also contain zinc which is important for healing wounds and making many of the body's processes function properly and which can be in short supply in toddlers' diets. Beans, peas and lentils are high in fibre so, if your child is eating these very often, avoid giving too many other wholegrain foods such as brown rice, wholemeal bread and pasta. Too much fibre can interfere with the absorption of calcium and iron and fill up small tummies so that it is difficult to get enough calories and nutrients.

'I've got eighteen quid a week for the food and that's it. You don't get much choice for eighteen quid. I know what I'd like to give the family to eat, and I know what I can afford to give them, and they're nothing like the same.'

'When you go shopping, your mind's on anything but shopping. You can't stop and think. You grab what you can and get out quick.'

Healthy fast food

Fruit and vegetables

Wholemeal bread or toast

Baked beans

Baked potatoes

Fish fingers and frozen fish generally – but grilled or baked rather than fried

Canned fish

Canned tomatoes

Natural yoghurt

Cooked eggs

Wholegrain breakfast cereals – which don't have to be eaten just as breakfast.

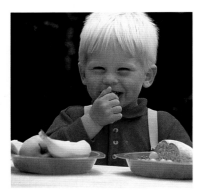

BETTER SNACKS

Fresh fruit

Raw vegetables like carrots

Natural yoghurt with fresh fruit

Chunks of cheese

Unsweetened breakfast cereals (dry or with milk)

Bread

Unsweetened biscuits

Popping corn

Bread sticks

'A lot of it is habit. I mean, if your children have never had sugar on their cereal in the morning, then they don't expect it. But then you mustn't have it either. The thing is that I like sweet things myself. In fact, at the moment, the more tired I get, the more I want to eat biscuits and that sort of thing. But if I eat them, the children eat them. The only answer is not to buy them in the first place.'

Bread, other cereals and potatoes

This group of starchy foods includes potatoes, sweet potatoes and yams, rice, pasta and noodles, maize and millet, breakfast cereals and all types of bread. They should form the main part of each meal, and they make cheap, nutritious and easily prepared snacks.

Starchy food provides energy, vitamins, minerals and fibre too. You can introduce one or two wholegrain varieties (such as wholemeal bread, brown rice or wholemeal pasta) early on and add more as your child gets older. It is not a good idea to only give wholegrain foods because they may fill your child up too quickly to get enough calories and nutrients.

Try to use unsweetened breakfast cereals and don't add bran to cereals or use bran-enriched cereals because the bran can interfere with the body's ability to absorb iron.

Fruits and vegetables

Fruits and vegetables are ideal first foods for babies as they contain vitamins and minerals and purée easily. As children become older fruits and vegetables make good finger foods and their different colours, textures and tastes make a toddler's meal interesting. They also contain fibre which helps prevent constipation, so try to make sure your child has at least four servings of fruits and vegetables each day.

Different fruits and vegetables contain different vitamins and minerals so the wider the range the better, but don't worry if your child will only eat one or two types. Allow him or her to eat them as often as possible and gradually tempt him or her with new varieties. If you can, try to include some green vegetables (broccoli, cabbage), and some yellow or orange vegetables (swede, carrots, squash) and fruit (apricots, peaches, mangoes). These contain beta-carotene, the plant

form of vitamin A. Also try to include some citrus fruits (satsumas, oranges) and some salad (tomatoes, peppers) for vitamin C.

Fruits, vegetables or juice high in vitamin C help iron to be absorbed from other foods, so give some at each meal. (See the box on page 71 for good sources of vitamin C.)

Many children don't like cooked vegetables but may nibble on them whilst you are preparing a meal. Be imaginative about serving vegetables, perhaps mashing different types together, or arranging them attractively on the plate (for example, carrot 'stepping stones' amongst the broccoli 'trees'). Encourage your child to eat fruit if they won't eat vegetables. Dried fruits such as apricots, prunes and peaches are a useful snack or can be made into puddings. Cut up apples, carrot and cucumber for snacks instead of sweets. If your child doesn't like fruit or vegetables, it is sensible to make sure he or she has vitamin drops.

FOODS CONTAINING SUGAR

Children are born with a taste for sweet things. Breast and formula milk taste sweet so they naturally prefer sweet flavours. However, we don't actually need sugar and giving your toddler sweet foods such as biscuits, cakes, lollies, fizzy drinks, squash and sweets will fill him or her up and spoil the appetite for healthier food. They can also damage the teeth.

This doesn't mean you should never give sweet foods, but try to make them occasional rather than daily foods. Sweet foods are best eaten in one go rather than over the course of an hour or two. Keep them for after mealtimes as a treat. Try to stick to milk or water for drinks. Squashes, fizzy drinks, colas and even fruit juice contain sugars

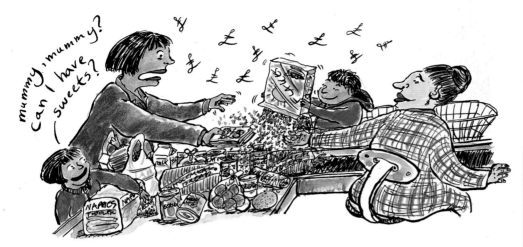

'Everybody knows that sweets aren't good. But they love them. And the fact is, it's a pleasure to treat them.'

which can cause tooth decay. Fizzy drinks are also acidic and excessive consumption can cause tooth erosion. The diet (reduced calorie) drinks, sweetened with artificial sweeteners such as saccharin, do not cause decay but are not suitable either. See Drinks pages 72–73.

Fruits and vegetables contain sugar in their cells. When the sugar is bound up in this way it is much less damaging to teeth, so try to use fruits and vegetables as alternative snacks to sweets and biscuits. Bread or unsweetened breakfast cereals (don't add sugar at the table) are good too. Look at the labels on foods; sugar may be listed as glucose, sucrose, honey, dextrose, maltose or syrup. If sugar is near the top of the ingredients list, then it's the largest or nearly the largest ingredient.

FOODS CONTAINING FAT

Children under the age of two need fat to supply them with a

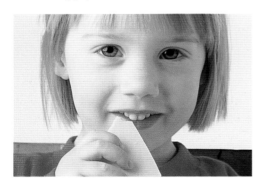

concentrated source of energy. Using full-fat milk, cheese, yoghurt, oily fish and butter will supply them with a good source of fats. Limit fatty foods such as crisps, biscuits, cakes or fried foods as eating too many of these can start bad eating habits for life. Between the ages of two and five you can gradually introduce lower fat dairy products and cut down on fat in other foods so that, by the time children are five, they are eating a low fat diet like adults.

Because fat is such a concentrated source of energy it is easy to eat too much of it and become overweight. It is a good idea to be aware of the amount of fat contained in foods which the whole family eat and to try to keep it to a minimum. Some ideas for cutting down on fat are shown in the box.

THE IMPORTANCE OF IRON

Iron is a vital mineral, used for making healthy blood. Babies are born with a supply of iron which lasts about six months, and after that they must eat foods which are a good source of iron to meet their needs. A baby who doesn't get enough iron can develop anaemia, which can hold back his or her development.

If babies have infant formula or follow-on milk as their main drink

---

TRY SOME OF THESE IDEAS FOR CUTTING DOWN FAT IN YOUR FAMILY MEALS

- *Grill or bake food instead of frying it. If you do fry, use an unsaturated oil like rapeseed, blended vegetable, olive, soya, sunflower or corn oil.*

- *Skim fat off meat dishes, like mince or curry, during cooking.*

- *Take the skin off poultry before cooking. The skin's the fattiest part.*

- *Trim the visible fat off red meat.*

- *Use vegetables or soaked dried beans with just small amounts of meat in stews and casseroles.*

- *Use low-fat spread or a margarine high in unsaturates rather than butter, hard margarine, or ordinary soft margarine (but not for children under two).*

- *Use lower fat cheese like one of the low-fat Cheddars, Edam, or cottage cheese (but not for children under two).*

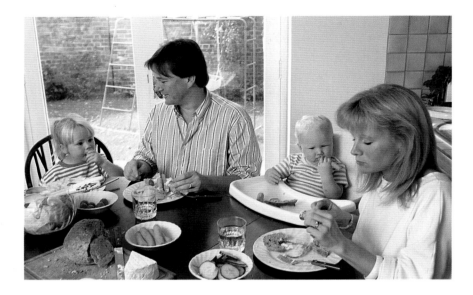

A little salt or sodium chloride is needed by the body, but it is possible to get all we need from foods without adding any more at the table or in cooking. Some salt is added to bread and cheese during production and other foods, such as bacon, ham, salami, crisps, savoury snacks, are high in salt. Toddlers do not need added salt and too much can lead to a liking for salty flavours and raised blood pressure in later life.

Try to limit the amount of salty foods your child eats and don't add any salt in cooking. The whole family will benefit if you reduce the amount of salt in cooking.

after six months, they will be getting some iron. But breastfed babies will need to rely more heavily on foods for iron after four to six months. All babies need a mixture of foods that provide iron.

There are two types of iron – one is found in meat and is easily absorbed by the body, and one is found in plant foods and is more difficult for the body to absorb. If foods containing vitamin C or meat or fish are eaten at the same meal, the plant type of iron is better absorbed. However tea, coffee and bran prevent iron being absorbed, so don't give these to your toddler, especially if they are having a vegetarian diet at mealtimes.

FOOD ADDITIVES

Foods contain additives for a variety of reasons – to prevent food poisoning, to stop foods from going off, to provide colour, flavour or texture. Some food additives are natural substances, others are synthetic, but the fact that it is natural does not make it 'better'. Any additives put into food must, by

GOOD SOURCES OF IRON	OTHER SOURCES OF IRON
	The iron in these is better absorbed if vitamin C, meat or fish is also given
canned sardines, pilchards, mackerel, tuna	*fortified breakfast cereals*
	dark green vegetables
	breads
liver paté, liver or kidney	*beans and lentils*
	tofu, hummus
lean beef, lamb or pork	*dried fruit; apricots, figs, prunes, peaches*
chicken or turkey (dark meat best)	

law, be shown on the label. Many are shown by the European Community 'E number'. Additives with E numbers have been tested and passed as safe for use in EU countries. Numbers without an E in front are allowed in the UK, but not in all EU countries.

A few people suffer from allergic reactions to some additives, but many more people are allergic to ordinary foods such as milk or soya. A diet which is high in processed foods is not only likely to contain additives, but will probably be higher in salt, sugar and fat than is desirable for adults and children. Replacing these foods with more fruits and vegetables and starchy foods is good advice.

FOOD ALLERGIES

Some children experience unpleasant reactions after eating certain foods. They might be sick, have diarrhoea, cough or wheeze or get an itchy rash, but they often outgrow these food sensitivities. However, some foods may cause a reaction so severe that it is life-threatening. Thankfully this affects very few children.

The foods most likely to cause a problem for small children and babies are often the ones they first meet at weaning. So it is sensible to avoid giving these foods until a baby is at least six months old. These foods include nuts and sesame seeds, wheat, fish, soya (unless soya-milk formula is advised by a doctor), citrus fruits (such as oranges) and eggs.

Serious allergies to nuts, nut products and some seeds affect less than 1 per cent of the population. For those who are at risk (people with a family history of hayfever,

asthma and eczma), it may be best to avoid these foods. Peanut allergy is a particular concern. For children at risk of peanut allergy, the advice is to avoid giving peanuts and foods containing peanut products, e.g. peanut butter, **unrefined** ground-nut oil and some snacks, until at least 3 years of age. Read food labels carefully and if you are still in doubt about the contents, these products should be avoided.

If you notice a pattern of adverse reactions in your child after he or she has eaten certain foods then your GP should be consulted. If necessary your child can then be referred to a dietitian or medical specialist.

Do not restrict your child's diet or cut out foods on the basis of unproven tests, or without expert advice on how to keep your child's meals properly balanced. This could be harmful to a small child who might still be eating a limited range of foods.

If you suspect your child may be susceptible to food allergic reaction, contact your GP who can refer the child to a specialist clinic. The National Asthma Campaign Helpline (0345 010203) can be contacted for advice, and so can The British Allergy Foundation. Their address is: Deepdene House, 30 Bellegrove Road, Welling, Kent DA16 3PY. Telephone: 0181 303 8525.

PROBLEMS WITH EATING

It can be a great worry if your child refuses to eat or is terribly choosy, but it is extremely rare for a child to actually starve him or herself. Children will eat enough to keep them going. So try not to worry unless your child is clearly not gaining weight as he or she should (see pages 37-38), or is obviously unwell.

It may be that your child is picking up your own feelings about food. Perhaps you're a dieter or have a weight problem, or maybe you just see healthy eating as a very important goal. If your child is picking up on your anxiety it may be that mealtimes have become an ideal time to get attention.

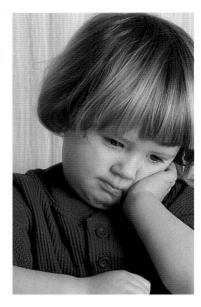

Just as anxiety may cause problems with toilet training, it can also create problems with eating. So try to take a step back and think about how much of a problem there really is.

REFUSING TO EAT, OR EATING VERY LITTLE

- **Don't force your child to eat.**

- **Don't leave meals until your child is overtired or too hungry.**

- **If your child refuses food or just picks at his or her food for a long time, call an end to the meal.** Do it calmly and not in anger, no matter what time and effort you've put into the cooking.

- **Put less on your child's plate and praise your child for eating even a little.**

- **Try to make meals enjoyable and not just about eating.** Sit down and chat about things other than food.

- **If your child prefers drinks to food, cut down on the amount of drinks you give just before meals.** You may even need to cut down on the milk drinks.

- **If you know other children of the same age who are good eaters, ask them to tea.** A good example sometimes works, so long as you don't go on about how good the other children are.

- **Ask another adult whom your child likes to eat with you.** Sometimes a child will eat for, say, a grandparent without any fuss. It may be only one meal out of many, but it could break a habit.

- **Your child may just be a naturally slow eater,** and so lots of patience will be needed.

- **Limit snacks and drinks between meals.**

- **Don't get trapped into giving your child a sweet treat after an uneaten meal.** A cake instead of fish fingers might be just what your child wants, but it's not going to help establish a sensible and nutritionally balanced eating pattern.

- **Children's tastes change.** One day they'll hate something and a month later they'll love it. There'll nearly always be enough that your child is willing to eat for some variety (say beans, fish fingers and fruit, and milk to drink). It may be boring, but it's perfectly healthy.

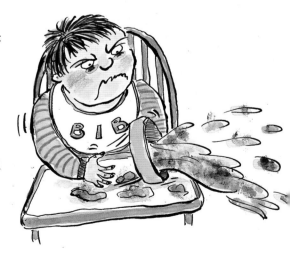

6 Illness and accidents

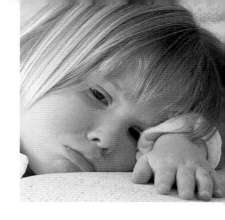

Every child gets ill occasionally and every parent has had that feeling of anxiety as they see their normally cheerful child looking sad and listless. Most bouts of illness pass quickly and leave children better able to resist the next attack. Sometimes, if the illness or accident is serious, immediate (and possibly long-term) help is needed. This chapter deals with common childhood illnesses and accidents, the best ways to prevent them, and the action to take in an emergency.

KNOWING WHEN YOUR CHILD IS ILL

Sometimes there's no doubt. But often it's difficult to tell whether a child is ill. Children may be listless, hot and miserable one minute, and running around quite happily the next. Watch out for:

- **some sign of illness** (like vomiting or a temperature, cough, runny nose, runny eyes);

- **behaviour that's unusual for your child** (like a lot of crying, being very irritable or refusing food and drink, being listless or drowsy).

Possible signs of illness are always more worrying if your child is a baby or very small. To know when to consult the doctor about your baby, see the box.

If your child is older and you're not sure whether or not to see the doctor, you might want to carry on normally for a while and see whether the signs of illness or pain

continue. It might be best not to let your child see you watching. Most children can put on an act, especially if they see you're worried.

Above all, trust your feelings. You know better than anyone what your child is like day-to-day, so you'll know what's unusual or worrying. If you're worried, contact your doctor. Even if it turns out that nothing is wrong, that is exactly what you need to know.

If you have seen your GP or health visitor and your baby isn't getting better or is getting worse, contact your GP again the same day. If you become worried and you can't get hold of your GP or your GP can't come to you quickly enough, then take your baby straight to the Accident and Emergency department of the nearest hospital, one with a children's ward if possible. It's worth finding out in advance where this is, in case you ever need it.

If you're seriously worried and/or know your child needs urgent attention, phone your GP at any time of the day or night. There may be a different number for when the surgery is closed. If you can't contact a GP, go directly to the nearest Accident and Emergency department. See inside the back cover for what to do in an emergency.

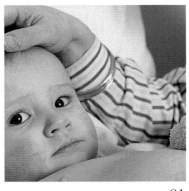

SICK BABIES —
ALWAYS CONTACT
YOUR DOCTOR IF:

● *you think your baby's ill,
even if you can't make
out what's wrong;*

● *your baby has one or more
of the problems listed in the
box below.*

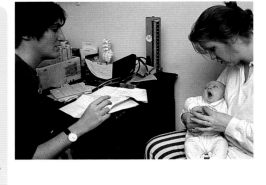

USING YOUR GP

*'He doesn't seem to listen. I'm
in and out in no time, and I
come home no better off than if
I'd stayed at home. In fact,
sometimes it makes it worse,
because he'll give me something
and I'll not know whether it's
really needed or not.'*

*'My doctor gives me advice.
He's also a Moslem, you see,
so he can give me advice about
any questions I want to ask.
He said if I had any
worries, I could always
go and talk to him.'*

Most practices are very supportive
towards parents of small children.
Many will fit babies into surgeries
without an appointment, or see them
at the beginning of surgery hours.
Many doctors will give advice over
the phone. Others will feel that it is
essential to see your child.

Some GPs are less helpful and it's
not always easy to phone or to get to
the surgery. Even so, if you're
worried about a particular problem
that won't go away, it's right to
persist. (See page 125 for information
on how to change your GP.)

Your health visitor and/or clinic
doctor can give you advice and help
you decide whether your child is
really unwell or not. But it's only
your family doctor (your GP) who
can treat your child and prescribe
medicines. If you think your child is
ill, it's best to see your GP.

If you're unsure whether to go to
the surgery or ask for a home visit,
phone and talk to the receptionist or
to your GP. Explain how your child is
and what's worrying you. Often it
doesn't do a child (or anyone else)
any harm to be taken to the surgery,
and you're likely to get attention
more quickly this way. But explain if
it's difficult for you to get there.
Wrapping a sick child up and going
by car is one thing; going on the bus
might be impossible.

USING MEDICINES

Medicine isn't always necessary
when your child is ill. Some
illnesses simply get better by
themselves and make your child
stronger and better able to resist
similar illness in the future. If you're
offered a prescription, talk with your
GP about why it's needed, how it
will help, and whether there are
any alternatives.

● When a medicine is prescribed,
ask about any possible side-effects.
Could it, for example, make your
child sleepy or irritable?

● Make sure you know how much
and how often to give a medicine.
Write it down if need be. If in doubt,
check with your pharmacist or GP.

● Always finish a prescribed course
of medicine. A course of antibiotics,
for example, usually lasts at least
five days. This is to make sure all
the bacteria are killed off. Your
child may seem better after two or
three days, but the illness is more
likely to return if you don't finish
all the medicine.

● If you think your child is reacting
badly to a medicine, for example
with a rash or diarrhoea, stop
giving it and tell your GP.
Keep a note of the name of the
medicine so you can tell your
GP in the future.

SYMPTOMS AND SIGNS THAT ARE ALWAYS URGENT:

● *a fit (convulsion), or if your baby turns blue or very pale (in a dark-
skinned baby check the palms of the hands) or seems floppy;*
● *a very high temperature (over 39 °C), especially if there's a rash;*
● *difficulty breathing, breathing fast or grunting breathing;*
● *unusually drowsy or hard to wake or doesn't seem to know you;*
● *a temperature, but the skin of the hands and feet feels cold and clammy;*
● *a purple-red rash anywhere on the body — this could be a sign of
meningitis (see photo on page 94).*

- If you buy medicines at the pharmacist, always say it's for a young child. Give your child's age. Some medicines are for adults only. Always follow the instructions on the label or ask the pharmacist if you're unsure.

- Ask for sugar-free medicines if they are available.

- Look for the date stamp. Don't use out-of-date medicines. Take them back to the pharmacy to be destroyed.

- Only give your child medicine given by your GP or pharmacist.

  Never use medicines prescribed for anyone else.

- Keep all medicines out of your child's reach and preferably out of sight – in the kitchen where you can keep an eye on them, rather than the bathroom.

- In the past, all medicines for children have been diluted to the right strength for each child with a liquid solution so that you could give it to your child on a 5 ml spoon. Now most medicines prescribed by your GP will no longer be diluted in this way. Instead you'll have to measure the correct dose for your child's age. The instructions will be on the bottle.

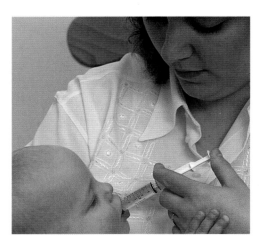

- Medicines that aren't diluted in liquid may need to be given using a 'liquid medicine measure', which looks like a syringe. It allows you to give small doses of medicine more accurately.

Always read the manufacturer's instructions supplied with the measure, and always give the exact dose stated on the medicine bottle. Some medicines will come with a measure supplied by the manufacturer, in which case that's the right measure to use. If in doubt ask the pharmacist for help.

LOOKING AFTER A SICK CHILD

It doesn't matter if your child doesn't want to stay in bed. Being with you, maybe tucked up in an armchair or on a sofa, might be less lonely. Children are usually sensible about being ill and if they say they're well enough to be out of bed, they very probably are.

- Don't overheat the room your child is in. Keep it airy without being draughty.

- See pages 90-91 for what to do if your child has a temperature.

- Give your child plenty to drink. For the first day or so don't bother about food unless it's wanted. After that, try to find ways of making a bit of food tempting.

- Try to give your child time for quiet games, stories, company and comfort.

- Sick children are often easily tired and need lots of rest. Encourage your child to doze off when he or she needs to, perhaps with a story read by you or on tape.

See pages 90-91 for what to do if your child has a temperature.

SYMPTOMS AND SIGNS THAT ARE SOMETIMES SERIOUS:

- *a hoarse cough with noisy breathing;*

- *crying for an unusually long time or in an unusual way or seeming to be in a lot of pain;*

- *refusing feeds;*

- *diarrhoea or vomiting, particularly both together;*

- *unusually hot or cold or listless or more drowsy than normal.*

Aspirin shouldn't be given to children under 12. It has now been linked with a rare but dangerous illness. Seek advice from your GP before taking aspirin if you are breastfeeding.

Paracetamol is safer, but don't give it to children under three months without asking your GP first. Make sure you've got the right strength for your child. Overdosing is dangerous. Read the label and/or check with your pharmacist.

Ibuprofen made for children can be given for pain and fever to children over the age of one who weigh more than 7 kg. Avoid if your child has asthma unless advised by your GP. Check the correct dose for your child's age. Don't give adult ibuprofen to children under the age of 12.

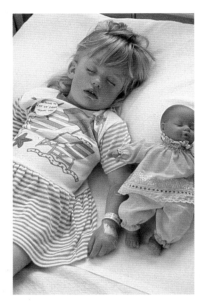

Looking after a sick child, even for a couple of days, is exhausting. Make things as easy for yourself as you can. Get rest and sleep when you can, and try to get somebody else to take over every now and then to give you a break.

CHILDREN IN HOSPITAL

Hospitals can be strange, frightening places for children. Being ill or in pain is frightening too. There's no parent who isn't anxious to do all they can to help their child.

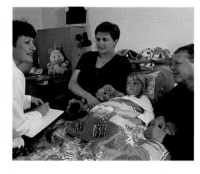

- **Prepare your child as best you can.** You could play 'doctors and nurses' or 'operations' with teddies and dolls and read story books about being in hospital. It's worth doing this even if you don't know your child is going into hospital. Quite a large number of under fives do have to go into hospital at some stage, and many go in as emergencies.

- **Be with your child in hospital as much as possible.** It's extremely important for you to be with your child in hospital as much as possible and, with young children especially, to sleep there. Do all you can to arrange this. All hospital children's departments now have some provision for parents to stay overnight with their children. Talk to hospital staff beforehand and be clear about arrangements, what will happen, and so on. You may then be able to explain at least a part of it to your child.

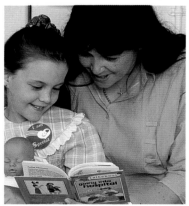

- **Explain as much as possible to your child.** Even quite young children need to know about what is happening to them, so explaining as much as possible is important. What children imagine is often worse than reality. Be truthful, too. Don't, for example, say something won't hurt when it will. Some hospitals will arrange visits for children and their families before the child is admitted for a planned treatment or operation.

- **Talk with hospital staff about anything that will be important for your child.** You may need to explain cultural differences. Staff should know, for example, if hospital food is going to seem very strange to your child. Try to discuss ways of getting over problems like this. Also tell staff about any special words your child uses (such as needing to go to the lavatory), any special ways of comforting, and so on.

- **Make sure something like a favourite teddy bear or comforter goes into hospital with your child.**

- **Be prepared for your child to be upset by the experience,** and maybe to show it in one way or another for some time afterwards. Reassure as much as you can.

You can get a lot of helpful information and advice on how best to cope when your child is in hospital from Action for Sick Children (address on page 134).

COMMON COMPLAINTS

SMOKING AND CHILDHOOD ILLNESSES

Children who live in a smoky atmosphere are more likely to get:

- coughs and colds

- chest infections (temperature with a bad cough)

- asthma

- ear infections and glue ear.

Every year 17,000 children are admitted to hospital because their parents smoke. If you can't stop smoking or encourage other adults in your house to stop, then try and make sure that your children don't have to smoke too by creating a smoke-free zone. See page 116 for tips on giving up.

ASTHMA

Asthma is an inflammatory condition of the airways (bronchial tubes) of the lungs. These carry the air we breathe. With asthma the airways are extra sensitive to substances or trigger factors which irritate them, such as dust, animal fur or cigarette smoke. When in contact with a trigger factor, the air passages become narrower and a sticky mucus (phlegm) is produced making it difficult for air to pass through. Asthma is on the increase, especially in children.

The exact cause of asthma is unknown, but an attack can be due to sensitivity (allergy) to a trigger factor or to non-allergic causes. It is known that asthma often runs in families.

Symptoms of asthma include

- Repeated attacks of coughing and wheezing, usually with colds, shortness of breath and production of phlegm. The symptoms are often worse at night or after exercise. Not everyone with asthma gets all the symptoms. And for many young children, a dry irritating cough may be the only symptom. See your GP if you think your child has asthma.

- Smoking during pregnancy or around a child, can increase the child's risk of asthma.

- Breastfeeding your child for as long as possible can help protect against asthma developing.

COLDS

It may seem that your child always has a cold or upper respiratory tract infection. In fact it is normal for a child to have a cold eight or more times a year. This is because there are hundreds of different viruses and young children are meeting each one of them for the first time. Gradually they build up immunity and get fewer colds.

- Colds are caused by viruses, not bacteria, so antibiotics don't help.

- Sometimes babies who are snuffly can't breathe easily when feeding or asleep. Raising the head of the mattress slightly by putting a blanket underneath may help. Your GP may prescribe nose drops, which can help. Nose drops should not, however, be used for more than a few days otherwise they may make the situation worse. Or you could try gently tickling your baby's nostrils with some cotton wool – a sneeze might help to clear your baby's nose.

- A menthol rub or capsules containing a decongestant liquid, which you can put on to clothes, or a cloth, may help your child breathe more freely, especially at

ANTIBIOTICS

Many doctors are now reluctant to prescribe antibiotics for common illnesses such as colds, or may adopt a 'wait-and-see' policy to make sure an infection is caused by bacteria. Not only are antibiotics ineffective against viruses, but inappropriate use of these can result in the child developing a resistant infection in the future. If your child is prescribed antibiotics, always make sure the course if finished, even if your child seems better.

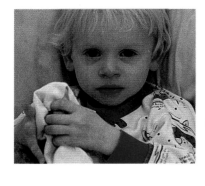

night. You can buy them from most pharmacists. You can also buy vaporisers, which can be helpful, but are expensive. Don't use menthol products for babies under three months without asking your GP, and be careful not to let your baby swallow a menthol capsule.

COUGHS

- Children may also cough when they have a cold because of mucus trickling down the back of the throat. If your child is feeding, eating and breathing normally and there is no wheezing, a cough is not usually anything to worry about. But if your child has a bad cough that won't go away, see your GP. If your child has a temperature and cough and/or is breathless, this may indicate an infection on the chest. If the cause is bacteria and not a virus, your GP will prescribe antibiotics to treat this – although it won't soothe or stop the cough straightaway.

- If a cough continues for a long time, especially if it is more troublesome at night or is brought on by your child running about, it might be a sign of asthma. Some children with asthma also have a wheeze or some breathlessness. If your child has any of these symptoms, he or she should be seen by your GP. If your child seems to be having trouble breathing, contact your GP, even in the middle of the night.

- Although it is distressing to hear your child cough, in fact, coughing serves a purpose. When there is phlegm on the chest, or mucus from the nose runs down the back of the throat, coughing clears it away. Most doctors

believe cough mixtures do not work and are a waste of money. To ease your child's cough, give him or her plenty of warm, clear fluids to drink. If your child is over the age of one, try a warm drink of lemon and honey. There is no need to try to stop the cough completely.

- **Croup is a result of infections that cause swelling at the back of the throat, along with difficulty in breathing.** Your child will have a hoarse cough and noisy breathing. Contact your GP if you think your child has croup. Sometimes, though not often, croup can be life-threatening. Therefore, it is important to watch out for danger signals like:

  - indrawing between the ribs or below the ribs with breathing
  - restlessness and lots of saliva
  - irritability
  - blueness of the lips or face.

If you notice any of these signs, call your GP or, if a doctor is not available, take your child straight to the nearest hospital with an Accident and Emergency department.

- If your child has croup a steamy atmosphere helps to relieve a 'croupy' cough and ease breathing. If your child has an attack of croup sit with him or her in the bathroom with the hot tap running or in the kitchen with water boiling. But be careful: very hot water, even if it isn't boiling, can scald. Keep the door and windows closed.

DIARRHOEA

YOUNG BABIES

Diarrhoea means frequent watery motions and is very common in babies. However, if the diarrhoea continues for more than a few hours, your baby will need extra

fluids. If you think your baby is also unwell, or if the watery motions go on for more than 24 hours, you should ask for your doctor's advice without delay.

- Your health visitor will be able to give you advice on feeding and on what extra fluids you should give and how often. There are special fluids available for this purpose which can be bought or prescribed by your doctor (for example Dioralyte, Rehydrate, Dextrolyte and Electrolade). If you are breastfeeding, continue to do so; in addition, give your baby the special fluids by bottle, cup or teaspoon. If you bottle feed your baby you should stop feeding for up to 24 hours, but make sure you give your baby enough of the replacement fluid. Your baby will take as much fluid as he or she needs, unless unwell.

Remember, if your baby is unwell, or if watery diarrhoea has lasted more than a day, seek your doctor's advice straight away.

OLDER CHILDREN
Contact your GP if your child is vomiting at the same time, or if the diarrhoea is particularly watery, has blood in it or goes on for longer than two or three days.

- Otherwise diarrhoea isn't usually worrying – just give your child plenty of clear drinks to replace the fluid that's been lost, but only give food if it's wanted. Do not give anti-diarrhoeal drugs unless prescribed by your GP.

- Help to prevent any infection spreading by using separate towels for your child and by reminding everyone in the family to wash their hands after using the toilet and before eating.

EAR INFECTIONS

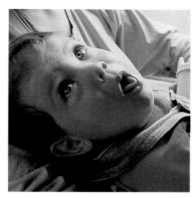

Ear infections are common in babies and small children. They often follow a cold and sometimes cause a bit of a temperature. Your child may pull or rub at an ear, but babies can't always tell where pain is coming from and may just cry and seem unwell and uncomfortable.

- If your child has earache but is otherwise well, paracetamol can be given for 12–24 hours. A covered hot water bottle can also be placed under your child's ear for warmth.

- Do not put any oil or eardrops into your child's ear unless advised by the GP.

- Some doctors prefer to treat ear infections with antibiotics, others feel the infection will clear up with paracetamol and decongestant nose drops.

After an ear infection your child may have a hearing problem for two to six weeks. If the problem persists after this time you should see your GP for further advice.

GLUE EAR

Repeated bouts of middle ear infections (called otitis media) may lead to 'glue ear' (otitis media with effusion). Here sticky fluid builds up and can affect your child's hearing. Your child may also have behaviour problems. If you smoke, your child is more likely to develop glue ear and will not get better so quickly. It is also better if your baby can be weaned from a bottle on to a cup. Your GP will give you further advice about the treatment for glue ear.

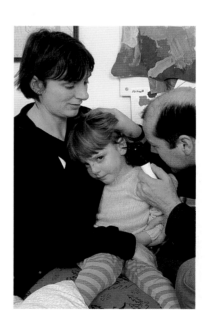

ECZEMA

Atopic eczema (which occurs mainly where there is a family history of eczema, asthma or hayfever) is thought to affect one in eight children. It often starts between the ages of two and four months with patches of red, dry and irritable skin on the face or behind the ears, and in the creases of the neck, knees and elbows. It can be very itchy. This can lead to your baby scratching and the eczema may sometimes become infected.

● If you think your child has eczema, speak to your GP or health visitor who may advise the use of creams or bath oils. In some cases, topical steroids may be needed for short periods.

● Avoid using substances that can dry or irritate your baby's skin such as baby bath, soap and detergents. Apply a moisturising cream or emollient to the skin several times a day (try to do this every time you change your baby's nappy or feed your baby).

● Keep your baby cool and avoid wool and nylon clothing; cotton is best.

● In some cases, allergens such as house dust mites, furry pets, cigarette smoke and chemicals may make the eczema worse.

FITS OR CONVULSIONS

Febrile convulsions or 'fever fits' are common in children under the age of three, but can seem very alarming to parents. Although there are other reasons why children 'fit', fits are most commonly triggered by a high temperature. If your baby or child seems feverish or has a high temperature it is important to cool him or her down immediately. See **Temperatures** on page 90–91 to find out how to do this.

What to do if your child has a fit

If your child has a fit he or she may suddenly turn blue and become rigid and staring. Sometimes the eyes will roll and the limbs start to twitch and jerk.

● Keep calm.

● Lie your child on his or her side to make sure he or she does not vomit or choke. Remove any objects from your child's mouth. Do not put anything in the mouth.
● Remove your child's clothing and any covering, and ensure your child is cool but not chilly.
● Sponge your child with tepid water if possible, starting from the head and working downwards.

Most fits will stop within three minutes. When it is over, reassure your child, make him or her comfortable, and then call a doctor.

● If the fit hasn't stopped, dial 999, or get someone else to go for help. Carry your child with you if there is no one to help you. If your GP isn't immediately available take your child to a hospital or call an ambulance. Stay with the child to prevent injury and move objects away from where the child is lying.

● Tell your GP that your child has had a fit.

Febrile convulsions become increasingly less common after the age of three and are almost unknown after the age of five. Children with *epilepsy*, which cause fits or seizures, may also grow out of these.

HEAD LICE

Head lice are tiny insects and are slightly smaller than a match

head. They can be difficult to see. Lots of children get head lice. It makes no difference whether their hair is clean or dirty. They catch them just by coming into contact with someone who is infested. When heads touch, the lice simply walk from one head to the other. They cannot jump or fly.

Signs of head lice

- A rash on the scalp.

- Lice droppings (a black powder, like fine pepper, may be seen on pillowcases).

- Eggs/nits – the lice lay eggs that are dull and well camouflaged, and hatch after about seven to ten days. Nits are the empty eggshells, about the size of a small pinhead. They are white and shiny and may be found further down the scalp, particularly behind the ears. They may be mistaken for dandruff but unlike dandruff, they're firmly glued to the hair and cannot be shaken off.

- Head itching – this is not always the first sign. Lice have usually been on the scalp for three or four months before the head starts to itch or they may not cause itching.

Checking for head lice

Lice are most easily detected by fine toothcombing really wet hair. Wet your child's hair and part it about 30 times. Comb each section carefully with a plastic, fine tooth nit comb. This should be done over a pale surface such as a paper towel or white paper, or over a basin of water or when your child is in the bath. Any lice present may be seen on the scalp or the comb, or may fall on the paper or in the water. They are usually grey or brown in colour.

Treatment of head lice

There are two ways of dealing with the problem.

'Wet combing' or non-insecticide method

- Wash the hair in the normal way with an ordinary shampoo.

- Using lots of hair conditioner and while the hair is very wet, comb through the hair from the roots with a fine tooth comb. Make sure the teeth of the comb slot into the hair at the roots with every stroke.

- Clear the comb of lice between each stroke with a tissue or paper towel.

- Wet lice find it difficult to escape, and the hair conditioner makes the hair slippy and harder for them to keep a grip, so that removal with the comb is easier.

- Repeat this routine every three to four days for two weeks so that any lice emerging from the eggs are removed before they can spread.

Lotions

Lotions and rinses that are specially made to kill lice and their eggs are available. If you choose to use these they can be bought from pharmacists. Your school nurse, health visitor or pharmacist will advise you which one to use. The lotion is changed frequently as the lice become resistant to it and it no longer works. If you cannot afford the lotion your GP may give you a prescription. **Follow the instructions carefully and *never* use these as a preventative measure.** The lotion kills the lice and nits, but the nits don't wash off. If you want to remove the nits you can buy a special nit comb from your pharmacy.

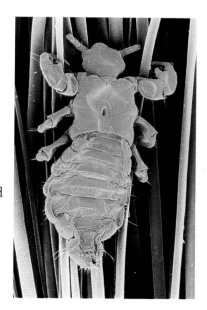

- *Shake down the mercury in the thermometer.*
- *Hold your child on your knee and tuck the thermometer under his or her armpit.*
- *Hold your child's arm against his or her body, and leave the thermometer in place for at least five minutes. It may help to read a story or watch television while you do this.*

NORMAL BODY TEMPERATURE

- *Under the arm, normal temperature is slightly lower than under the tongue – about 36.4 °C (97.4 °F).*
- *Under the tongue, normal temperature is about 37 °C (98.4 °F), but may vary a bit.*

STRIP–TYPE THERMOMETERS

Strip-type thermometers, which you hold on your child's forehead, are not an accurate way of taking temperatures. They show the skin and not the body temperature.

EAR THERMOMETERS

A digital thermometer is put in the child's ear. They take the temperature in one second and do not disturb the child, but are expensive.

Remember

- One infected child can infect an entire nursery – so do treat your child as soon as you discover head lice.

- Tell the nursery and other parents.

- Check your child's hair regularly, and always check if there is an outbreak at the nursery or school.

- If your child has head lice, check the whole family (including dad!) and treat them if necessary.

- Older people, such as grandparents, may have head lice without knowing it and may pass these on to children.

- Brush and comb your child's hair often – it helps prevent head lice taking hold.

NAPPY RASH
See page 25.

SORE THROAT

Many sore throats are caused by viral illnesses like colds or flu. Your child's throat may be dry and sore for a day or so before the cold starts.

Sometimes a sore throat is caused by tonsillitis. Your child may find it hard and painful to swallow, have a high temperature, and swollen glands at the front of the neck, high up under the jaw.

The majority of sore throats will clear up on their own after a few days. Paracetamol can be given to help the pain.

If your child has a sore throat for more than four days, has a high temperature and is generally unwell or is unable to swallow fluids or saliva, see your GP.

TEETHING
See page 33.

TEMPERATURES

BABIES UNDER SIX MONTHS

Always contact your GP if your baby has other signs of illness (see box on page 82) as well as a raised temperature and/or if your baby's temperature is 39 °C or higher.

If the doctor doesn't find a reason for the temperature, he or she will almost certainly want to send a urine specimen to the laboratory. A detailed test will show if your baby has a urine infection.

OLDER CHILDREN

A little fever isn't usually a worry. **Contact your GP if your child seems unusually ill, or has a high temperature which doesn't come down.**

- It's important to encourage your child to drink as much fluid as possible. Cold, clear drinks are best. Even if your child isn't thirsty, try to get him or her to drink a little and often, to keep fluids up. Don't bother about food unless it's wanted.

Bringing a temperature down
This is important because a continuing high temperature can be very unpleasant and, in a small child, occasionally brings on a fit or convulsion (see page 88).

- Take off a layer of clothing or bedclothes.

- Undress your child to his or her nappy or underclothes and vest and take off the bedclothes or just cover with a sheet.

- Try sponging your child's body, arms and legs with tepid water. Don't dry the skin. As the water evaporates, it takes heat out of the body.

- Paracetamol or children's ibuprofen if your child is over the age of one (make sure it's the right strength for your child), will also help to lower the temperature.

- Give cool drinks.

- Don't wrap your child up.

- Make sure the room isn't too hot.

VOMITING

BABIES

Babies often sick up a bit of milk, some a lot, without distress. But if your baby is vomiting often or violently and/or there are other signs of illness, contact your GP straightaway.

Your baby can lose a dangerous amount of fluid if he or she is sick often, especially if your baby has diarrhoea as well. See under **Diarrhoea** for how to make sure your baby is getting enough fluid.

OLDER CHILDREN

Older children can be sick once or twice without any bother and be well again quickly afterwards, or after a night's sleep. If your older child goes on vomiting, and/or there are other signs of illness, contact your GP.

- Give your child plenty to drink – clear drinks rather than milk. Don't bother about food unless he or she wants it.

THREADWORMS

Many children get threadworms. They spread by producing large numbers of tiny eggs which cannot be seen with the eye. The eggs are present in dust and stick to food, carpets, towels, bedlinen and toilet seats. Because they are so small and widespread they get on fingers and under finger nails and are easily swallowed. In the bowel they hatch into worms, which lay eggs around the bottom. You'll see them in your child's stools, looking like tiny white threads. Your child may have an itchy bottom and may scratch it a lot, especially at night.

If you think your child has worms, see your GP or health visitor, or ask your pharmacist for treatment. Everybody in the family has to be treated because the threadworm eggs spread very easily.

To prevent the infection spreading

- Keep your child's nails short.

- Let your child wear pyjamas or pants in bed.

- Bath your child or wash around the bottom each morning.

- Keep your child's towel separate.

- Make sure everyone in the family washes their hands and scrubs their nails before every meal and after going to the toilet.

- Disinfect the toilet seat, toilet handle or chain regularly.

- Vacuum and dust bedrooms thoroughly.

SPOTTING A RASH

Rashes look different on different people. The colour of spots can vary and, on a black skin, rashes may be less easy to see. If in doubt, check with your GP. Small children and babies sometimes get rashes that are not due to infectious illnesses and which soon go without treatment. For information about meningitis and septicaemia see page 94.

HEPATITIS B

If you'd like to know more about Hepatitis B virus or Hepatitis B immunisation, your health visitor or GP will be happy to talk to you.

ILLNESS	INCUBATION PERIOD (The time between catching an illness and becoming unwell)	INFECTIOUS PERIOD (When your child can give the illness to someone else)
CHICKEN POX	11–21 DAYS	From the day before the rash appears until all the spots are dry.
MEASLES	7–12 DAYS	From a few days before the rash appears until 5 days after it goes.
MUMPS	14–21 DAYS	From a few days before becoming unwell until swelling goes down. Maybe 10 days in all.
RUBELLA (GERMAN MEASLES)	14–21 DAYS	One week before and at least 4 days after the rash first appears.
WHOOPING COUGH	7–14 DAYS	From the first signs of the illness until about 6 weeks after coughing first starts. If an antibiotic is given, the infectious period is up to 5 days after beginning the course of treatment.

Begins with feeling unwell, a rash and maybe a slight temperature. Spots are red and become fluid-filled blisters within a day or so. Appear first on the chest and back, then spread, and eventually dry into scabs, which drop off. Unless spots are badly infected, they don't usually leave a scar.

No need to see your GP unless you're unsure whether it's chickenpox, or your child is very unwell and/or distressed. Give plenty to drink. Paracetamol will help bring down a temperature. Baths, loose comfortable clothes and calamine lotion can all ease the itchiness. You should also inform the school/nursery in case other children are at risk.
Keep your child away from anyone who is, or who is trying to become, pregnant. If your child was with anyone pregnant just before he or she became unwell, let that woman know about the chicken pox (and tell her to see her GP). Sometimes chickenpox in pregnancy can cause miscarriage or the baby may be born with chicken pox.

Begins like a bad cold and cough with sore, watery eyes. Child becomes gradually more unwell, with a temperature. Rash appears after third or fourth day.

Spots are red and slightly raised; may be blotchy, but are not itchy. Begins behind the ears, and spreads to the face and neck and then the rest of the body. Children can become very unwell, with cough and high temperature.
The illness usually lasts about a week.

See your GP. If your child is unwell give him or her rest and plenty to drink. Warm drinks will ease the cough. Paracetamol will ease discomfort and lower the temperature. Vaseline around the lips protects the skin. Wash crustiness from eyelids with warm water.

At first, your child may be mildly unwell with a bit of fever, and may complain of pain around the ear or feel uncomfortable when chewing. Swelling then starts under the jaw up by the ear. Swelling often starts on one side, followed (though not always) by the other. Your child's face back to normal size in about a week. It's rare for mumps to affect boys' testes (balls). This happens rather more often in adult men with mumps. For both boys and men, the risk of any permanent damage to the testes is very low.

Your child may not feel especially ill and may not want to be in bed. Baby or junior Paracetamol will ease pain in the swollen glands. Check correct dosage on pack. Give plenty to drink, but not fruit juices. They make the saliva flow, which can hurt. No need to see your GP unless your child has stomach ache and is being sick, or develops a rash of small red/purple spots or bruises.

Can be difficult to diagnose with certainty. Starts like a mild cold. The rash appears in a day or two, first on the face, then spreading. Spots are flat. On light skin, they are pale pink. Glands in the back of the neck may be swollen. Your child won't usually feel unwell.

Give plenty to drink. Keep your child away from anybody you know who's up to 4 months pregnant (or trying to get pregnant). If your child was with anyone pregnant before you knew about the illness, let her know. If an unimmunised pregnant woman catches German measles in the first 4 months of pregnancy, there is a risk of damage to her baby.
Any pregnant woman who has had contact with German measles should see her GP. The GP can check whether or not she is immune, and if not, whether there is any sign of her developing the illness.

Begins like a cold and cough. The cough gradually gets worse. After about 2 weeks, coughing bouts start. These are exhausting and make it difficult to breathe. Your child may choke and vomit. Sometimes, but not always, there's a whooping noise as the child draws in breath after coughing. It takes some weeks before the coughing fits start to die down.

If your child has a cough that gets worse rather than better and starts to have longer fits of coughing more and more often, see your doctor. It's important for the sake of other children to know whether or not it's whooping cough. Talk to your GP about how best to look after your child and avoid contact with babies, who are most at risk from serious complications.

MENINGITIS AND SEPTICAEMIA

These symptoms may not all appear at the same time. In babies look for the following:

- *A high-pitched, moaning cry.*
- *The baby being difficult to wake.*
- *Refusing to feed.*
- *Pale and blotchy skin.*
- *Red or purple spots anywhere on the body that do not fade under pressure – do the 'Glass Test' (see below).*

In older children look for the following signs:

- *Red or purple spots that do not fade under pressure – do the 'Glass Test' (see below).*
- *Stiffness in the neck – can the child kiss his or her knee, or touch his forehead to the knee?*
- *Drowsiness or confusion.*
- *A severe headache.*
- *A dislike of bright light.*

The 'Glass Test'

*Press the side or bottom of a glass **firmly** against the rash – you will be able to see if the rash fades and loses colour under the pressure. If it doesn't change colour, contact your GP immediately. (See photo below.)*

If your child becomes ill with one or more of these signs or symptoms, contact your GP urgently. You may be asked to go straight to the surgery or the nearest Accident and Emergency Department.

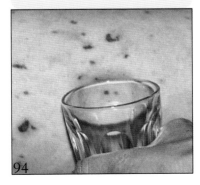

INFECTIOUS ILLNESSES

MENINGITIS AND SEPTICAEMIA– WHAT TO LOOK FOR

Meningitis is an inflammation of the lining of the brain. It is a very serious illness, but if it's picked up and treated early, most children make a full recovery. **Septicaemia** is blood poisoning, which may be caused by the same germs that cause meningitis. Septicaemia is also very serious and must be treated straightaway.

In recent years there has been a lot of concern about meningitis in children. There are several different types of meningitis. The Hib vaccine gives protection against **Hib meningitis** but it doesn't protect your child against other bacterial types, such as **meningococcal** or **pneumococcal** or **viral meningitis**.

The early symptoms of meningitis such as fever, irritability, restlessness, vomiting and refusing feeds are also common with colds and flu. A baby with meningitis or septicaemia can become seriously ill within hours. Some of the symptoms, such as a severe headache, are difficult to see in babies because they cannot tell you how they feel. The important signs to look out for are shown in the box to the left. **If your child has a red or purple rash, look at it through a glass tumbler. The meningitis rash does not blanch (that is fade or turn white) when the bottom or side of the tumbler is pressed firmly against it, whereas almost all other childhood rashes do. If you can't get in touch with your GP, or if you are still worried after getting advice, trust your instincts – take your child to the nearest Accident and Emergency department.**

IMMUNISATION

IMMUNISATION IS THE SAFEST AND MOST EFFECTIVE WAY OF PROTECTING YOUR CHILD AGAINST SERIOUS DISEASES

Your child should have their first immunisation when he or she is 2 months old. Your health visitor, practice nurse or GP will make an appointment with you, or they will send you an appointment inviting you to bring your child for immunisation. Most surgeries and health centres run special immunisation or baby clinics and there is often a 'drop in' facility at other times for parents who can't get to the clinic during the day. Remember all chilhood immunisations are free.

COMMON QUESTIONS ABOUT IMMUNISATION

What is immunisation and how does it work ?

Immunisation prepares our bodies to fight against diseases in case we come into contact with them in the future. For example, immunisation against polio stimulates the immune system to produce antibodies against polio. If your child ever comes into contact with polio, the polio antibodies will recognise the disease and be ready to fight it.

Babies are born with some natural immunity which they get from their mother and through breastfeeding. This gradually wears off as the baby's own immune system starts to develop. Having your child immunised gives extra protection against illnesses which can kill.

Does immunisation last for ever?

Some immunisations have to be given more than once to build up immunity (protection) or keep the level of antibodies topped up. This 'top up' is called a booster.

How are immunisations given and do they hurt?

All immunisations, except polio, are given with a small needle into the upper arm, thigh or buttock. Children may cry and be upset for a few minutes, but they usually settle down after a cuddle. If you don't want to be in the room when your child has the injection, tell the nurse or doctor beforehand. Some parents find it helpful to take a friend or partner to hold the child during the injection.

Are there any reasons why my child should not be immunised?

There are very few reasons why a child should not be immunised. **You must let your health visitor, doctor or nurse know if your child:**

- has a high fever;

- has had a bad reaction to another immunisation;

- has had, or is having, treatment for cancer;

- has a bleeding disorder – one that some children get is called ITP;

- has had a **severe** reaction after eating eggs; or

- has had convulsions (fits) in the past. (With the right advice, children who have had fits in the past can be immunised.)

You should also let your health visitor, doctor or nurse know if your child or any other close family member:

- has any illness which affects the immune system, for example, HIV or AIDS; or

- is taking any medicine which affects the immune system, for example, immunosuppressants (given after organ transplant or for malignant disease) or high-dose steroids.

How do we know that vaccines are safe?

Before any vaccine can be used it has to go through many tests. Research from all over the world shows that vaccines are the safest way of protecting your child's health. Each vaccine is continually checked after it has been introduced and action is taken if it is needed. If a vaccine is not safe it is not used.

How will my child feel after immunisation?

All children are different. Most will not be affected. Sometimes redness and swelling may develop where the injection was given. But do not worry, it will slowly disappear. A few children may be unwell and irritable and develop a temperature.
Very rarely, children can have allergic reactions straight after immunisation. If the child is treated quickly, he or she will recover fully. People giving immunisations are trained to deal with allergic reactions.

How do I know if my child has a fever and what should I do?

If your child feels hot to touch and looks red or flushed, he or she probably has a fever (a temperature over 37.5°C). You can check this with a thermometer.

Treat a fever by doing the following:

- Keep your child cool by gently sponging him or her with lukewarm (**not** cold) water. Let the water dry on the skin.

95

- Make sure your child does not have too many layers of clothes or blankets on.

- Give your child extra drinks.

- Give your child Paracetamol liquid, such as Calpol, Disprol or Medinol. Read the instructions on the bottle carefully and give the dose according to your child's age. For babies it is helpful to use a special medicine syringe so you can measure the dose accurately. Ask your pharmacist for one. If necessary, give your child a second dose 4 to 6 hours later. If their temperature is still up, ask your doctor for advice.

Do not give aspirin to children under 12 years of age.
- Some health visitors, practice nurses and doctors may tell you to give your child a dose of Paracetamol when you get home after an immunisation. In many cases this will prevent your child developing a fever.

You don't hear about most of the diseases we vaccinate against now, so is immunisation really necessary?
These diseases still exist in many parts of the world and there are still cases in this country. If your child is not immunised, he or she is still at risk.

Immunisation doesn't just protect your child and your family, it protects the whole community, especially those children who can't be immunised.

By immunising as many people as possible, fewer people will catch diseases. So the diseases will get rarer and rarer. With effective immunisation programmes, some diseases, for example, polio, mumps and measles, will disappear.

WHEN SHOULD I CALL THE DOCTOR?

*Contact your GP **immediately** if your child has a temperature of 39 °C or above or has a fit. If the surgery is closed and you can't contact the duty doctor go to your nearest hospital Accident and Emergency department.*

Follow your instincts and speak to your doctor if you are worried about your child.

CHILDHOOD IMMUNISATIONS

DTP-Hib VACCINE

This is given when your child is 2, 3 and 4 months old. (The DT part is also given at age 3 to 5 years as a booster.)
The DTP-Hib vaccine protects against three different diseases: **Diphtheria**, **Tetanus** and **Pertussis** (whooping cough) and against infection by the bacteria called Haemophilus influenzae type b (Hib).

Your child will receive a further tetanus and diphtheria booster at age 13 to 18 years.

What is diphtheria?
This disease begins with a sore throat and can progress rapidly to cause problems with breathing. It can damage the heart and the nervous system and in severe cases it can kill. Diphtheria has almost been wiped out in the UK, but it still exists in other parts of the world and it is on the increase in parts of Eastern Europe.

What is tetanus?
Tetanus germs are found in soil. They enter the body through a cut or burn. Tetanus is a painful disease that affects the muscles and can cause breathing problems. If it is not treated, it can kill.

And what about whooping cough (pertussis)?
Whooping cough can be very distressing. In young children it can last for several weeks. Children become exhausted by long bouts of coughing which often cause vomiting and choking. In severe cases pertussis can kill.

I hadn't heard of Hib before, what is it?
Hib is an infection that can cause a

number of serious illnesses including blood poisoning, pneumonia and meningitis. All of these diseases can be dangerous if not treated quickly. The Hib vaccine protects your child against this one specific type of meningitis. The Hib vaccine does not protect against any other type of meningitis. For information about other types of meningitis see page 94.

How effective is Hib vaccine?

Before the Hib vaccine became part of the childhood immunisation programme in 1992, over 60 children a year died as a result of Hib infection. And more than twice that number were left with permanent brain damage. Since immunisation began, the number of children with Hib meningitis has dropped by more than 95%.

What are the side effects of the DTP-Hib vaccine?

It is quite normal for your baby to be miserable within 48 hours of the injection. Some babies develop a fever in the way described earlier. Sometimes a small lump develops where the injection was given. This lump can last for several weeks.

If your child has a worse reaction to the DTP-Hib vaccine – for example, some form of fit – your doctor may not give your child any more doses of the vaccine. If this happens, talk to the doctor, nurse or health visitor.

If a baby has a fit in the first 48 hours after being given the DTP-Hib vaccine at 2, 3 and 4 months, it is no more common than at any other time for young babies. But if you delay the immunisation, it increases the chances of fits after DTP-Hib. So, it's important to make sure your child gets vaccinated on time.

Is it true that the whooping cough vaccine can cause brain damage?

In the 1970s a study was done which seemed to show a link between the whooping cough vaccine and a few babies who suffered brain damage. More recent and reliable studies have not confirmed this theory. But the actual whooping cough disease can cause brain damage.

POLIO VACCINE

This is given when your child is 2, 3 and 4 months. The first booster is given when your child is between 3 and 5 years. The second booster is given when your child is between 13 and 18.

Polio vaccine protects against the disease **poliomyelitis**.

What is polio?

Polio is a virus that attacks the nervous system and can cause permanent muscle paralysis. If it affects the chest muscles it can kill. The virus is passed in the faeces (poo) of infected people or those who have just been immunised against polio. Routine immunisation has meant that the natural virus no longer causes cases of polio in the UK. But polio is still around in other parts of the world, especially in India.

How is it given?

Unlike other immunisations, you take the polio vaccine by swallowing it. The doctor or nurse drops the liquid into your child's mouth.

Are there any side effects?

There is an extremely small chance of developing polio from the imm-unisation – the risk is of one case in more than 1.5 million doses used.

The nurse at the clinic told me to be careful about changing my child's nappy after the immunisation. Why is this?

The polio vaccine is passed into your child's nappies for up to six weeks after the vaccine is given. If someone who has not been immunised against polio changes your child's nappy, it is possible for them to be affected by the virus. There is about one case each year. This works out at about one case for every 1.5 million doses used. You must wash your hands thoroughly to prevent this happening.

If you think you have not had the polio immunisation, contact your doctor. You can arrange to have it at the same time as your child. This also goes for anyone else in the family who looks after your child.

MMR VACCINE

This is given when your child is between 12 and 15 months and then again when your child is 3 to 5 years.

The MMR vaccine protects your child against **Measles**, **Mumps** and **Rubella (German measles)**.

What is measles?

The measles virus is very infectious. It causes a high fever and a rash. About one in 15 children who gets measles is at risk of complications which may include chest infections, fits and brain damage. In severe cases measles can kill.

What is mumps?

The mumps virus causes swollen glands in the face. Before immunisation was introduced, mumps was the commonest cause of viral meningitis in children under 15. It can also cause deafness, and swelling of the testicles in boys and ovaries in girls.

What is rubella?

Rubella, German measles, is usually very mild and isn't likely to cause your child any problems. However, if a pregnant woman catches it in her early pregnancy, it can harm the unborn baby.

Do children really need protection against these illnesses? I've heard they're usually mild.

Yes, they can be mild. In some children the illness may pass almost unnoticed, but others can be very ill. The most dangerous thing about these illnesses is that they can cause complications.

Before the vaccine was introduced, about 90 children a year in the UK died from measles. Because of immunisation, children no longer die of measles.

Why are two doses of MMR given?

Your child will receive two doses because measles, mumps and rubella vaccines don't always work well enough on the first go. The second MMR immunisation makes sure that your child gets the best protection against these three diseases. This also gives a second chance for those children who missed out the first time around. So, you can be sure your child is well protected before they start school. Giving a second dose of MMR is a recent improvement to children's immunisation in the UK. Two doses are already used in this way in many countries including the USA and Canada.

What about children who are allergic to eggs?

The MMR vaccine is prepared in egg but it can be given to children who are allergic to eggs. If your child has had a **serious** reaction to eating eggs, or food containing egg, then talk to your doctor. The usual signs of a serious allergic reaction are a rash that covers the face and body, a swollen mouth and throat, breathing difficulties and shock. In these cases your doctor can make special arrangements for the immunisation to be given safely.

Are there any side-effects of the MMR vaccine?

About a week to 10 days after the MMR immunisation some children become feverish, develop a measles-like rash and go off their food for two or three days. Very rarely, a child will get a mild form of mumps about three weeks after the injection. Your child will not be infectious at this time, so they can mix with other people as normal.

Occasionally, children do have a bad reaction to the MMR vaccine. About one child in a thousand will have a fit. A child who actually has measles is **10 times** more likely to have a fit as a result of the illness. Although encephalitis (inflammation of the brain) has been reported very rarely after immunisation, the risk of children developing encephalitis after the measles immunisation is no higher than the risk of children developing encephalitis without the vaccine. But the risk of a child developing encephalitis after having measles is about one in 5000. And $1/3$ of these children will be left with permanent brain damage. A study of British children shows that 10 years after the measles immunisation, children had no more illnesses than children who had not been immunised – and actually had fewer because they were protected against measles and did not suffer its complications.

Your child may get a rash of small bruise-like spots after the MMR, but this is very rare. This rash is linked with the rubella part of the immunisation. If you see spots like this, show them to your doctor.

Side effects from the second MMR vaccine are even rarer than after the first. Those that do happen are most likely in children who did not respond to the first vaccine. These are the children who need the immunisation most. There are no new side effects of a second MMR vaccine.

OTHER IMMUNISATIONS

BCG VACCINE

This is given when your child is between 10 and 14 years. It is sometimes given to babies shortly after they are born.
The BCG vaccine gives protection against TB (tuberculosis).

What is TB?
TB is an infection that usually affects the lungs. It can also affect other parts of the body such as the brain and bones.

I didn't think you could get TB in this country.
Although TB is no longer common in this country, there are between 5,000 and 6,000 cases a year. TB is on the increase in Asia, Africa and some Eastern European countries.

When do children normally have the BCG vaccine?
Most children have the BCG injection when they are between10 and 14. Your child will have a skin test to see if they already have immunity to TB. If not, the immunisation is given. Babies under three months who are having the immunisation don't need to have the skin test.

Are there any side effects of the BCG immunisation?
A small blister or sore appears where the injection is given. This is quite normal. It gradually heals leaving a small scar.

HEPATITIS B VACCINE
This vaccine gives protection against **hepatitis B**.

What is hepatitis B?
There are several different types of hepatitis and they all cause inflammation of the liver. The hepatitis B virus is passed through

GOING ABROAD

Your child may need extra immunisations. Check, at least two months in advance, with your GP or travel clinic (look in your phone book).

infected blood and may also be sexually transmitted.

Some people carry the virus in their blood without actually having the disease itself. If a pregnant woman is a hepatitis B carrier, or gets the disease during pregnancy, she can pass it on to her child. The child may not be ill but has a high chance of becoming a carrier and developing liver disease later in life.

Can this be prevented?

Yes, many pregnant women are tested for hepatitis B during their ante-natal care.

Babies born to infected mothers should receive a course of vaccine to prevent them getting hepatitis B and becoming a carrier. The first dose should be given within two days of birth, and two more doses should be given before the child is six months.

Are there any side effects?

Side effects of the vaccine tend to be quite mild. The injection site is often red and can be sore for a few days afterwards.

If a mother has hepatitis B is it still safe to breastfeed?

Yes, you are still safe to breastfeed as long as the baby is immunised.

ALTERNATIVES TO
IMMUNISATION

Is immunisation voluntary?

In the UK parents can choose whether to have their children immunised. Children who are not immunised run a risk of catching diseases and having complications. Immunisation is the safest way to protect your child. Having children immunised at an early age means they are well protected by the time they start playgroup or school where they are in contact with lots of children. If you have any doubts or questions about immunisation, talk to your health visitor, practice nurse or doctor.

Can homeopathic vaccines protect against infection?

No, there is no proven, effective alternative to conventional immunisation. Homeopathic medicine has been tried as an alternative to the whooping cough vaccine but it was not effective. The Council of the Faculty of Homeopathy (the registered organisation for doctors qualified in homeopathy) advises parents to have their children immunised with conventional vaccines.

When is the immunisation due?	Which immunisations	Type	Date the immunisation is given
At two months	Polio	By mouth	
	Hib Diphtheria Tetanus Whooping cough	One injection	
At three months	Polio	By mouth	
	Hib Diphtheria Tetanus Whooping cough	One injection	
At four months	Polio	By mouth	
	Hib Diphtheria Tetanus Whooping cough	One injection	
At 12 to 15 months	Measles Mumps Rubella	One injection	
3 to 5 years (usually before the child starts school)	Measles Mumps Rubella	One injection	
	Diphtheria Tetanus	One injection	
	Polio	By mouth	

TRAVEL IMMUNISATIONS

Do children need extra immunisations if they are travelling abroad?

Children may need extra immunisations depending on their age, which country you are visiting and how long you plan to stay. You should contact your doctor or a travel clinic for up-to-date information on the immunisations your child may need. If you are travelling to an area where there is malaria, your child will need protection. This is one of the most serious health problems in tropical countries. There isn't an immunisation against malaria, but some anti-malarial drugs can be given to children. It is essential to do all you can to avoid getting bitten by mosquitoes. Insect repellent, mosquito nets soaked in repellent and making sure arms and legs are covered between dusk and dawn will all help. Be careful not to use too much repellent on your child's skin.

SAFETY

Accidents are the most common cause of death among children aged between one and five years.

Every year about 600,000 children under five go to hospital because of an accident in the home.

Children need to explore and to learn about the things around them. The safer you make your home, the less likely it is that their exploration will land them in hospital. Outside your home it's not so easy to make sure that the world is a safe place, but by getting together with other parents you can make a difference.

You can put pressure on your local council as follows:

- to make road crossings safer

- to mend stairs and walkways and improve lighting

- to clear rubbish tips and board up old buildings.

PROTECT AND TEACH

- **Under-threes** can't be expected to understand or remember safety advice. They need to have an adult nearby at all times.

- **Three-year-olds** can start learning how to do things safely, but expect your child to forget if she or he is excited or distracted.

- **Eight-year-olds** can usually remember and act on safety instructions, though they are not yet safe enough to cross a busy road alone. They need adults around to call on for help at all times.

- **Under eleven-years-old** children are unable to judge speed and distance, so they should never cross busy roads alone. From the age of eight or nine children could cross quiet roads alone but they must wait until there are no cars at all. They should know and understand the Green Cross Code.

SAFETY CHECKLIST

Use this list to check whether you're doing everything you can to prevent accidents. It's impossible to list all dangers, but thinking about some of these should start you thinking about others. Tick off the things you've done.

Danger – choking and suffocation

☐ Do you store small objects away from babies and small children who might put them in their mouths?

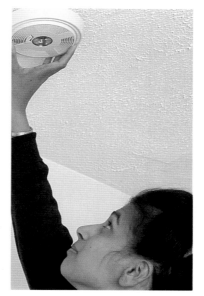

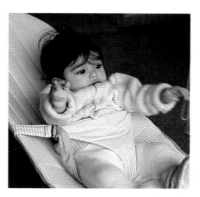

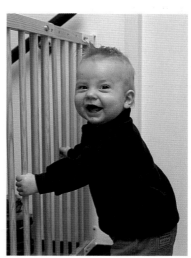

101

Have you got rid of ribbons and strings that might, either in play or by accident, get wound around a child's neck?

Do you keep peanuts away from children in your house? They often cause choking.

Do you store polythene bags out of children's reach?

Danger – fires, burns and scalds

Have you fitted a smoke detector?

Have you checked your smoke detector battery this week?

Could you get out of your house in a fire?

Have you shortened your kettle flex or bought a coiled flex? Dangling flexes from irons and kettles can be pulled.

Do you have a fire guard, fixed to the wall, round any kind of open fire (coal, gas or electric) or a hot stove?

Do you always use the back rings on the cooker and turn pan handles away from the front of a cooker? A flat work surface on either side of the cooker will prevent your child reaching pan handles at the side of the cooker. Or you could fit a cooker hob guard.

Do you use a playpen, cot or high chair (with restraints) to keep your child safe while you cook?

Do you keep your child away when you're drinking or carrying hot drinks and put mugs and cups, coffee jugs and teapots out of reach?

Have you put your tablecloths away? A child pulling at the edges can bring a hot drink or teapot down.

Do you always run the cold tap first in the bath and test the temperature before your child gets in? Be especially careful once your child is big enough to get into the bath without help and can play with the taps.

Have you turned down the hot water thermostat to 54 °C or 130 °F to avoid scalds?

Do you always cover hot water bottles to prevent burns and remove them from the bed before your child gets in?

Danger – falls

Do you always put bouncing chairs on the floor rather than a table or worktop?

Do you have a properly fixed stair gate or barrier, preferably at both the top and bottom of your stairs?

Baby walkers are dangerous. They tip babies down stairs and on to fires and radiators. Don't tick this box until you have thrown yours out.

Have you checked the rails round your landing and balconies? Could your child fall through, crawl under, climb over? Horizontal railings are especially dangerous.

Do you have safety catches or locks on your upstairs windows to stop your child falling out? Are you sure you won't be locked or nailed in if there is a fire?

Danger – cuts

Low-level glass in doors and windows is dangerous, especially once your child is on the move. Have you boarded it up, fitted safety film, or safety glass?

Do you keep all sharp things somewhere safe (away from children)?

Do you make sure your children never walk around holding anything made of glass or with anything like a pencil or lollipop stick in their mouths?

Danger – poisoning

☐ Have you locked all alcohol and medicines away or stored them high up, out of sight and where the child can't climb?

☐ Are your medicines in child-resistant containers? In other people's houses watch out for dangers like tablets in drawers and handbags.

☐ Are your household and garden chemicals in a safe place, high up, or locked away? Some chemicals are sold with child-resistant caps. Make sure you replace the cap properly after use.

☐ Are you sure there are no dangerous liquids in a bottle or jar that could make them look like drink?

☐ Are you teaching your children not to eat any plants, fungi, berries or seeds?

☐ If you use surma on your child's eyes, is it one of the safe, lead - free brands? Talk to your pharmacist. Some surma can be dangerous.

Danger – electricity

☐ Are your electric sockets covered by heavy furniture or safety covers when not in use?

☐ Have you repaired all worn flexes?

☐ Are you careful not to plug too many appliances into one socket?

Danger – drowning

☐ Do you know you should never leave a baby or young child under four alone in the bath for a moment? If the phone or doorbell rings, take your child with you, or let it ring.

☐ Is your garden pond covered or fenced off? Never leave your child alone near water.

☐ Does your child know how to swim? Children who can swim are safer, but it is still no guarantee of safety, so you should still keep a close watch when your children are near water.

Danger – cars

☐ Do you know the law?

● It's illegal to carry an unrestrained child in the front seat.
● It's illegal to carry an unrestrained child if there is a suitable restraint in the car.
● If there's a child restraint in the front but not in the back then children under three must use it.
● If there's an adult restraint in the front but not in the back children over three years must use it.
● You can only carry unrestrained passengers if there are more passengers than seat belts.

In general, it's safer for a child over three to use an adult belt than not to use a belt at all. Children should never be allowed to travel in the back of a hatchback (unless it has been specially adapted and fitted with seat belts) or to stand in a moving car.

☐ Do you have a rear-facing baby seat or a special restraint system for your carrycot?

☐ Do you have a child safety seat for toddlers?

☐ Do you have a booster cushion for bigger children to use with an adult safety belt?

☐ Do you always make sure you get your children out of the car on the pavement side?

☐ If you have air bags fitted to your car, do you make sure your baby always travels in the back seat?

In a growing number of areas there are loan schemes for baby safety seats. Through these schemes, you can get the seats more cheaply. Some schemes are run by local maternity hospitals. Or ask your midwife, health visitor, or road safety officer.

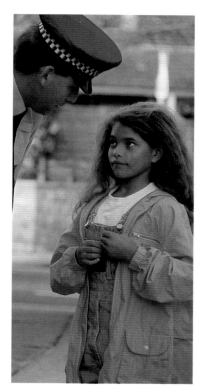

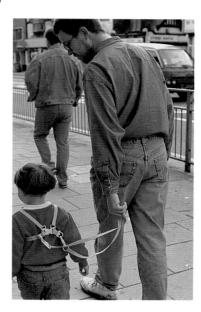

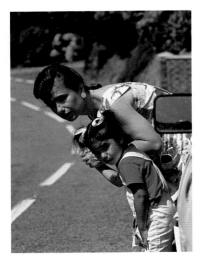

Danger – roads

- Never let a child on or near roads alone. Young children don't understand the danger of traffic.

- Hold your child's hand when you're near roads. Walking reins are useful for toddlers.

- Teach your child to cross roads safely by always crossing safely yourself and explaining what you're doing. Don't expect any child under the age of eight to cross a road alone.

Danger – strangers

Parents are often very worried about the possibility that their child will be abducted or murdered by a stranger. In fact this is a rare occurrence compared, for example, with the risk of a traffic accident. Nevertheless it's sensible to teach your children the following.

- Never go with anyone (even someone they know well) without telling the grown-up who is looking after them.

- If someone they don't know tries to take them away, it's OK to scream and kick.

- Tell your children always to tell you if they've been approached by someone they don't know.

- Make sure your child knows what to do if he or she is lost.

- In a crowded place, it's safest to stand still and wait to be found.

    Otherwise:
- tell a police officer

- go into a shop and tell someone behind the counter

- tell someone who has other children with them.

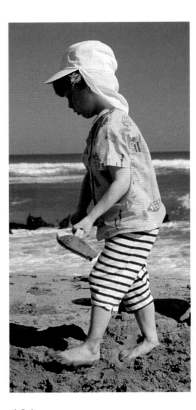

Teach your child his or her address and phone number or the phone number of some other responsible person.

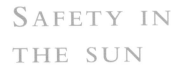

SAFETY IN THE SUN

The amount of sun your child is exposed to may increase his or her risk of skin cancer later in life. Do the following to protect your child.

- Keep your child out of the sun between 11 am and 3 pm when the sun is highest and most dangerous.

- Keep babies under the age of six months out of the sun altogether.

- Make the most of shade, such as trees.

- Don't let your child run around all day in a swimsuit or without any clothes on.

- Cover your child up in loose baggy cotton clothes such as an oversized T-shirt with sleeves.

- In particular, protect your child's shoulders and back of neck when playing, as these are the most common areas for sunburn

- Let your child wear a 'legionnaire's hat' or a floppy hat with a wide brim that shades the face and neck.

- Cover exposed parts of your child's skin with a sunscreen, even on cloudy or overcast days. Use one with a minimum sun protection factor (SPF) of 15 and which is effective against UVA and UVB. Re-apply often.

- Protect your child's eyes with sunglasses with an ultra-violet filter, made to British Standard 2724.

- Use waterproof sunblock if your child is swimming.

EMERGENCY FIRST AID

If, for whatever reason, you think your child may have stopped breathing, first you must make sure that it is safe for yourself and any other child to approach. Then you should try gently shaking and pinching your child and shouting 'wake up'. If you get no response from your child then he or she is unconscious and you must follow the **ABC of resuscitation** shown below. **You should also call for help**.

A OPEN THE AIRWAY

1 Place your child on a firm surface.
2 Look inside the mouth for any obvious obstruction which can be removed easily.
3 Put your hand on your child's forehead and gently lift the chin with two fingers.

Do not touch the back of the throat: young children's palates are very soft and may swell or bleed, further blocking the airway.

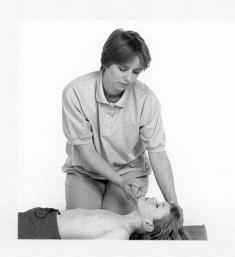

B CHECK BREATHING FOR AT LEAST 10 SECONDS

1 Put your ear close to your child's mouth.
2 Look to see if the chest is rising and falling.
3 Listen for sounds of breathing.
4 Feel for breath on your cheek.
5 Do this for 10 seconds

If your child is not breathing give five breaths of mouth to mouth ventilation (see page 106), then check circulation.

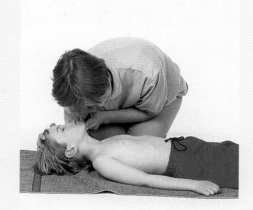

C CHECK CIRCULATION FOR AT LEAST 10 SECONDS

For babies (under one year)
Check the pulse inside the upper arm by lightly pressing two fingers towards the bone. Do this for 10 seconds.

For children (over one year)
Check the pulse in the neck by lightly pressing two fingers to one side of the windpipe.

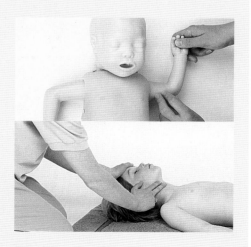

COPING WITH ACCIDENTS

You'll have to cope with some accidents while your child is young, mostly minor, but some may be major.

- *Learn basic first aid, or revise what you already know. There's information on the following pages. You can also buy books.*
- *Better still, do a first aid course. Courses are run by both the British Red Cross and St John Ambulance (the St Andrew's Ambulance Association in Scotland). These organisations have local branches. Look in your phone book, or contact the address on page 136 or ask your health visitor to organise a course.*
- *The Royal Life Saving Society UK arranges courses in baby resuscitation skills. If you would like to enquire about courses in your area, or would like further information, then telephone 01789 773994 or fax 01789 773995. A step-by-step emergency sequence leaflet* Save a baby's life *on the steps to take when a baby is choking or stops breathing is available from River House, High Street, Broom Warwickshire B50 4HN- please send a large stamped addressed envelope.*
- *Make sure you know what to do to get help in an emergency. See inside the back cover.*

IF YOUR CHILD HAS A PULSE
BUT IS NOT BREATHING

1 Start mouth to mouth
   ventilation (see below).
2 Continue for one minute, then
   carry your child to a phone and
   dial 999 for an ambulance, or
   get someone else to call for you.
3 Continue mouth to mouth
   ventilation. Check pulse
   every minute.

IF YOUR BABY OR CHILD HAS NO
PULSE AFTER FIVE SECONDS (OR
YOUR BABY HAS A PULSE SLOWER
THAN ONE BEAT PER SECOND) AND IS
NOT BREATHING

Start chest compression (see page
107) together with mouth to mouth
ventilation.

IF YOUR CHILD HAS A PULSE AND IS
BREATHING

1 Place your child in the
   recovery position (see page 107).
2 Dial 999 for an ambulance.
3 Check breathing and pulse
   frequently.

MOUTH TO MOUTH VENTILATION

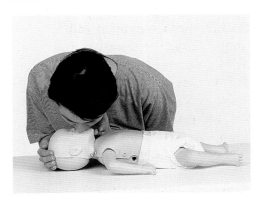 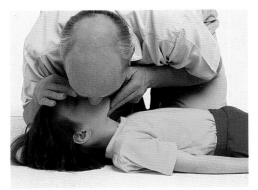

Babies (under one year)
1 Seal your lips around your
   baby's mouth and nose.
2 Blow gently, looking along the
   chest as you breathe. Fill your
   cheeks with air and use this
   amount each time.
3 As the chest rises, stop blowing
   and allow it to fall.
4 Do this at a rate of 20 breaths
   per minute.
5 Check pulse after 20 breaths.
   If present and above 60 beats
   per minute, continue mouth to
   mouth ventilation. If absent or
   below 60 beats per minute,
   commence chest compression.
6 If breathing starts, place your
   baby face down in your arms or
   lap with the head held low.

Children (over one year)
1 Seal your lips around your child's
   mouth while pinching the nose.
2 Blow gently, looking along the
   chest as you breathe. Take shallow
   breaths and do not empty your
   lungs completely.
3 As the chest rises, stop blowing
   and allow it to fall.
4 Do this at a rate of 20 breaths per
   minute.
5 Check pulse after 20 breaths.
   If still present continue mouth to
   mouth ventilation. If absent,
   commence chest compression.
6 If breathing starts, place
   your child in the recovery
   position.

CHEST COMPRESSION TOGETHER WITH MOUTH TO MOUTH VENTILATION

Note: Chest compression must always be combined with mouth to mouth ventilation.

Babies (under one year)

1 Place your baby on a firm surface.
2 Find the correct position – a finger's width below the nipple line, in the middle of the chest.
3 Use two fingers and press down on the chest by 2 cm ($3/4$ in.).
4 Press five times in about three seconds, then blow once gently into the lungs.
5 Continue for one minute.
6 Take your baby to a phone and dial 999, or get someone else to call for you.
7 Continue resuscitation (five compressions followed by one breath) until help arrives.
8 Only if colour improves check the pulse. If present, stop chest compressions but continue to give mouth to mouth ventilation if necessary.

Children (over one year)

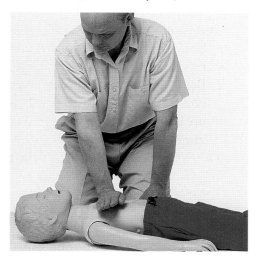

1 Place one hand two fingers' width above where the edge of the ribs meet the breastbone.
2 Use the heel of that hand and press down on the chest by 3 cm ($1 1/4$ in).

3 Press five times in about three seconds, then blow once gently into the lungs.
4 Continue this process for one minute.
5 Take your child to a phone and dial 999, or get someone else to call for you.
6 Continue resuscitation (five compressions followed by one breath) until help arrives.
7 Only if colour improves check the pulse. If present, stop chest compressions but continue to give mouth to mouth ventilation if necessary.

RECOVERY POSITION

The aim of the recovery position is to keep the airway open and minimise further injury.

Babies (under one year)

1 Don't use the recovery position.
2 Hold your baby face down in your arms or your lap, in each case with the head held low.

Children (over one year)

Note: For small toddlers it may be more practical to follow the guidelines for babies. Otherwise:

1 Place the arm nearest you at right-angles to the body, elbow bent. Bring the other arm across the chest. Hold the hand, palm out, against the cheek.
2 Roll your child on to his or her side, so that the upper leg is bent at the knee and the arms remain in the position described above.

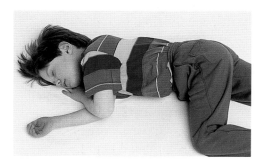

Don't give your child anything to eat or drink after an accident. Wait until you get to the hospital. He or she may need an anaesthetic later.

3 Tilt the head back gently to maintain the open airway.
4 If in the correct position, as shown, your child will not roll on to his or her tummy or back.
5 Check breathing and pulse. **If either stops, follow the ABC of resuscitation.**

IF YOUR CHILD HAS A BROKEN BONE

- Don't move your child if you think his or her neck or spine may be injured. Get expert help. Unnecessary movement could cause paralysis.

- A bone in your child's leg or arm may be broken if he or she has pain and swelling, and the limb seems to be lying at a strange angle.

- If you can't easily move your child without causing pain, call an ambulance.

- If you have to move your child be very gentle. Use both hands above and below the injury to steady and support it (using blankets or clothing if necessary). Comfort your child and take him or her to hospital.

IF YOUR CHILD IS BURNT OR SCALDED

- **Immediately** put the burn or scald under running cold water to reduce the heat in the skin. Do this for at least 15 minutes. If running water isn't possible, immerse the burn or scald in cold water or any other cooling fluid such as milk.

MINOR ACCIDENTS

Many general practices are equipped to deal with minor casualties such as cuts or items trapped in the nose or ear. In these sorts of cases therefore it may be more appropriate or convenient for you to seek advice from your local practice on where best to go, before attending an Accident and Emergency department.

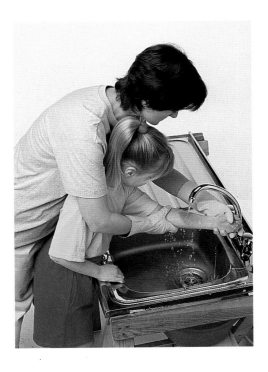

- Cover the burn or scald with a clean, non-fluffy cloth like a clean cotton pillow case or linen tea towel or cling film. This cuts down the danger of infection.

- If clothes are stuck to the skin, don't try to take them off.

- Depending on the severity of the burn or scald, see your doctor or call an ambulance or take your child to hospital. You should seek medical help for anything other than a very small burn.

- Don't put butter, oil or ointment on a burn or scald. It only has to be cleaned off again before treatment can be given.

- Don't prick any blisters. You'll delay healing and let in germs.

- Be prepared to treat your child for shock (see page 111).

IF YOUR CHILD IS CHOKING

Choking is caused by an obstruction in the airway and must be treated **immediately**.

- Look inside your child's mouth and remove any object if it is very easy to get at. Do not probe blindly into the mouth – you may push the object further in or damage the soft palate.

- If your child isn't breathing, start mouth to mouth ventilation – it may be possible to ventilate your child if the obstruction is only partial. If your child is breathing, follow the instructions below.

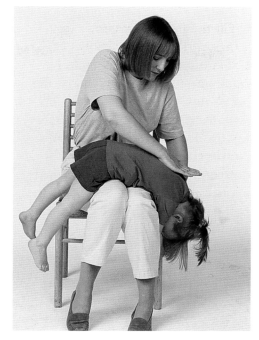

Babies (under one year)

1 Lie the baby along your forearm or thigh with the face down and the head low and supported.
2 Give up to five firm slaps between the shoulder blades.
3 If this does not work, turn your baby on his or her back along your thigh head down. Give five chest thrusts using the same technique and finger position as for chest compressions (see page 107), but press more sharply at a rate of about 20 per minute.
4 If this does not work, dial 999 and continue repeating the sequence of back slaps and chest thrusts.
5 **If your baby becomes unconscious follow the ABC of resuscitation (see page 105).**

> DO NOT USE ABDOMINAL THRUSTS ON BABIES UNDER ONE YEAR.

Children (over one year)

1 Encourage your child to cough if possible.
2 Bend your child forwards, so that his or her head is lower than the chest, and give up to five firm slaps between the shoulder blades.
3 If this does not work, lie your child on its back and give up to five chest thrusts using the same technique and finger position as for chest compressions (see page 107) but press more sharply at a rate of about 20 per minute.
4 If unsuccessful, give up to another five back slaps.
5 If this does not work, give **abdominal thrusts**. Place yourself behind your child and steady him or her with one arm. Put your other arm around your child, placing the heel of your hand in the upper abdomen. Give a sharp pull inwards and upwards below your child's ribs. Repeat up to five times.
6 If this does not work, summon medical aid and continue repeating the sequence of back slaps, chest thrusts, back slaps, abdominal thrusts.
7 **If your child becomes unconscious follow the ABC of resuscitation** (see page 105).

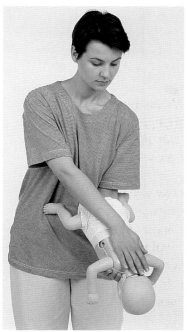

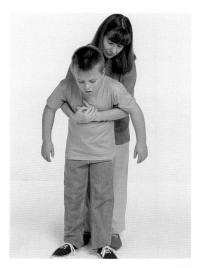

WHEN TO TAKE YOUR CHILD TO HOSPITAL AFTER AN ACCIDENT

- *If your child is unconscious*

- *If your child is vomiting or drowsy*

- *If your child is bleeding from the ears*

- *If your child has stopped breathing at some stage*

- *If your child may have internal injuries*

- *If your child complains of severe pain anywhere*

- *If your child is having fits (see page 88)*

If you're worried or uncertain about your child's injuries, get a doctor's advice. If you are unsure whether you should move your child, make him or her warm and call an ambulance. Go to the Accident and Emergency department of your nearest hospital or to a local doctor, whichever is quickest. Not all hospitals have an Accident and Emergency department, so check in advance where your nearest one is. Your health visitor will be able to tell you. (See inside the back cover for how to get help in an emergency.)

THINGS STUCK UP NOSE OR EARS

If you suspect that your child has stuck something up into his or her ear or nose, don't attempt to remove it yourself (you may push it further in). Take your child to the nearest Accident and Emergency department. If the nose is blocked explain to your child that he or she will have to breathe through the mouth.

IF YOUR CHILD HAS A CUT

- If there's a lot of bleeding, press firmly on the wound using a pad of clean cloth. If you don't have a cloth, use your fingers. Keep pressing until the bleeding stops. This may take 10 minutes or more.

- Don't use a tourniquet or tie anything so tightly that it stops the circulation.

- If possible, raise the injured limb. This helps to stop the bleeding. *But don't do this if you think the limb is broken.*

- Cover the wound with a clean dressing if you can find one. If blood soaks through the pad or dressing, do not remove it. Place

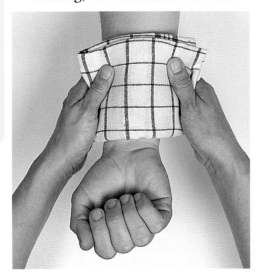

another pad or dressing over the top.

- Then call an ambulance or take your child to hospital.

- Ask your GP about a tetanus injection.

IF YOUR CHILD HAS TAKEN A POISON

Pills and medicines

- If you're not sure whether your child has swallowed something,

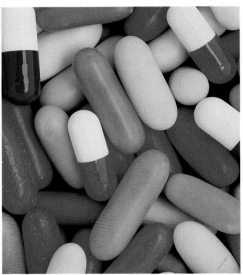

spend a minute or two looking for the missing pills. Check they haven't rolled under a chair, for example.

- If you still think something has been swallowed, take your child straight away to your GP or to hospital, whichever is quickest.

- Keep a close watch on your child and be prepared to follow the **ABC of resuscitation if he or she becomes unconscious** (see page 105).

- If possible, take the container (or its label) with you and a sample of whatever you think your child has swallowed.

- Don't give salt and water or do anything else to make your child sick.

Household and garden chemicals

- If you think something poisonous has been swallowed, calm your child as much as you can. You'll do this better if you can keep calm yourself. **But act quickly to get your child to hospital.**

- If possible, take the container (or its label) with you and a sample of whatever you think has been swallowed.

- If your child is in pain or there is any staining, soreness or blistering around the mouth, then he or she has probably swallowed something corrosive. Let him or her sip milk or water to ease the burning in the lips. Get your child to hospital quickly.

IF YOUR CHILD IS SHOCKED

- If pale, unwell or feeling faint after an accident, help your child to lie down.

- Keep your child covered up and warm, but not too hot.

- If your child has lost a lot of blood, keep his or her head down and raise your child's legs. This makes more blood go to his or her head. **But don't do this if you suspect a head injury or a broken leg.**

IF YOUR CHILD SUFFOCATES

- Quickly take away whatever is causing the suffocation.

- **If your child has stopped breathing, follow the ABC of resuscitation** (see page 105).

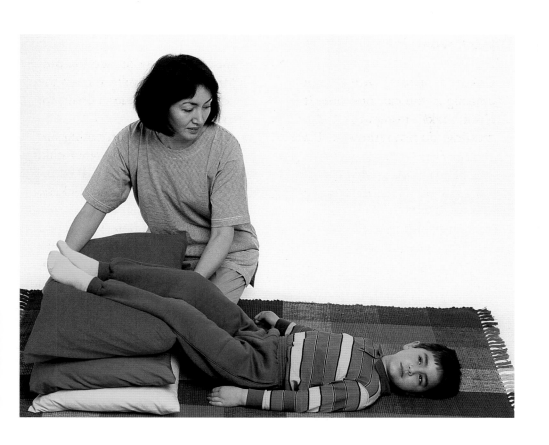

WHEN A CHILD DIES

'There was this huge emptiness, and the only way we could fill the emptiness and begin to understand was to talk and talk, and to cry. The real friends were the ones who let us talk and weren't afraid to see us cry. The last thing we wanted was to be helped to feel better. That would have meant forgetting what had happened to us before we'd even begun to live with it. It would have meant forgetting our baby. You never forget. It will always be part of us, just like any child.'

'Time goes by and gradually, if you grieve enough, you begin to accept it. A time comes when you can make it all right with yourself to feel happy about happy things.'

There's a feeling that children aren't meant to die. That feeling adds great shock (as well as maybe anger, bewilderment, even a kind of guilt) to the enormous grief and sadness brought by death. The grief, sadness and other feelings are important to you. They're not to be set aside quickly or hidden away.

You need to let yourself grieve in your own way. If you need to cry, don't hold back the tears. Crying may be the only way of letting out your feelings. If you feel angry, as many parents do, or find you're blaming yourself or others, it's important to talk about it. Ask the questions you want to ask of, for example, hospital staff, your GP, midwife, or health visitor. Often the reasons for a baby's death are never known, not even after a post-mortem. But you need to find out all you can.

After the first shock, it may help you to think about ways of remembering your child. If you don't already have photographs you may want to have a photograph

taken to keep. Talk to the hospital about this. Give a lot of thought to any service or ceremony you may want, and to mementoes you may want to keep.

Try to explain what's happened as simply and honestly as you can to any older children. They need to understand why you're sad, and will have their own feelings to cope with. Sometimes an older child connects the death with something he or she has done, and may be very quiet, or badly behaved, for a time. It's not easy for you to give the love and reassurance that's needed. It may help to get support from others close to your child.

Coping with the outside world and other people is difficult at first. You may find that even people quite close to you don't know what to say, say the wrong thing, or avoid you. Take the support that's given and feels right.

It's best to expect a long time of difficult feelings and ups and downs. Talking may not come easily to you, but even some time after your baby's death, it can help to talk about your feelings. The more you and your partner can talk to each other, the more it'll help you both. A father's experience of a baby's death can be different from a mother's. Although you'll share a lot, your feelings and moods won't be the same all the time. Try to listen to each other so you can support each other as best you can.

Sometimes talking to someone outside the family is helpful – a close friend, your doctor, health visitor, hospital staff, maybe a priest or other religious counsellor.

Talking to other parents who've been through the same loss and grief can be a special help. You can contact other parents through the following organisations.

- *The Stillbirth and Neonatal Death Society*
  Run by and for parents whose baby has died either at birth or shortly afterwards.

- *The Foundation for the Study of Infant Deaths*
  Supports parents bereaved by a cot death or what is called 'Sudden Infant Death Syndrome' (SIDS) .

- *The Compassionate Friends*
  An organisation of, and for, all bereaved parents.

Addresses and phone numbers are given on page 135

7 Your own life

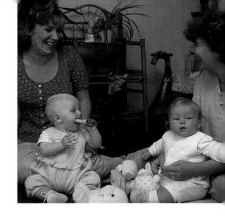

Becoming a parent changes your life. Suddenly there seems to be no time for you, for the things you liked to do, for quiet moments with your partner or with friends. Sometimes you may feel that there isn't even any time for the basic things in life like eating and sleeping. But if you don't give yourself some time and consideration, your batteries will soon be used up and you simply won't have the energy to make a good job of being a parent. This section is for you.

YOUR BODY AFTER CHILDBIRTH

Having a baby changes your body. You may not like the changes, or you may enjoy feeling different 'more like a mother'. If you like the way you are, don't let other people tell you different.

If you feel uncomfortable with your body you'll want to make some changes. Some things will never be quite the same again – for example, stretch marks will fade, but won't ever go away completely.

Other changes need not be permanent. A saggy tummy can be tightened up with exercise, and weight gain will gradually drop off if you eat and exercise sensibly. But don't expect any of this to happen overnight. It took nine months to make a baby. Give yourself at least that long to get back into shape again – and it may take longer.

In the meantime, give your body some little treats to cheer you up. For example, if it makes you feel good to paint your toe nails, then make time to do it. Maybe for you that's even more important than 20 minutes extra sleep.

'People say, "How's the baby doing?" And I want to say "Well she's OK, but do you want to know how I'm feeling?"

'I'm totally knackered, but I wouldn't give them back for anything!'

'I suppose I'd thought that having a kid wouldn't change that much for me. Obviously it was going to make a difference financially, with Linda giving up work. Apart from that, I'd thought it was Linda's life that was going to change and that I'd be going on much the same as before. Who was I kidding?'

(A FATHER)

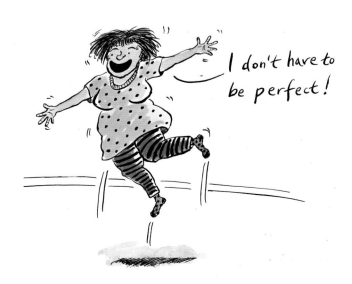

I don't have to be perfect!

PHYSICAL PROBLEMS

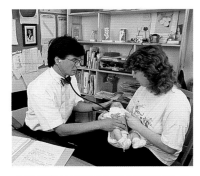

POSTNATAL CHECK

Don't be so busy looking after your baby that you forget to attend for your postnatal examination at around six to eight weeks. This is an opportunity for you to talk to your doctor about any health problems following delivery such as perineal pain or pain following episiotomy, backache, piles, incontinence etc. It is also an opportunity for you to talk about how you are feeling, for example if you are feeling low or depressed, and also to talk about family planning if you wish.

A lot of women have physical problems, either as a result of labour and birth, or because of the kind of work involved in caring for young children, or both. Problems like some sort of infection that keeps coming back, back pain, a leaky bladder and painful intercourse are much more common than people think. These sorts of problems can get you down, and some get worse if they're not seen to.

HELPING YOURSELF

For some problems you can do a lot to help yourself. The muscles around your bladder, vagina and back passage (the perineum) may be weak and that could be part of the reason for the 'falling out' feeling or leaky bladder that many women describe. Pelvic floor exercises can help. A bad back can also be helped by exercise, and by learning to use your back carefully.

Pelvic floor exercise
The muscles of the pelvic floor form a hammock underneath the pelvis to support the bladder, womb and bowel. You use these muscles when you pass water, empty your bowels and when you make love. Often they're stretched during pregnancy, labour and birth. If you can improve their strength and function you're less likely to have a leaky bladder, and more likely to enjoy intercourse.

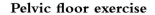

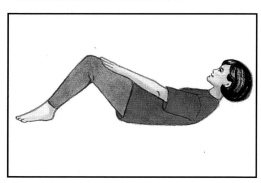

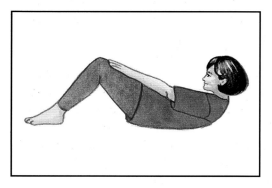

You can do this exercise either sitting or standing, when you're washing up, queuing in the supermarket, watching television – anywhere. You ought to do it for the rest of your life. It's an exercise that's just as important for older women as younger.

- Squeeze and draw in your back passage at the same time. Close up and draw in your vagina (front passage) upwards.

- Hold on for about five seconds, then let go.

- Do this exercise in sets of five, ten times a day.

It helps to imagine you're stopping a bowel movement, holding in a tampon, stopping yourself passing water. In fact, the best way to find the muscles is to try stopping and starting (or slowing down) the flow of urine while you're on the toilet.

Curl ups

This exercise firms up your stomach and closes the gap in the abdominal muscles that opens up during pregnancy.

- Lie on the floor (rather than your bed) with your knees bent up high so your feet are flat on the floor.

- Pull your tummy in and gradually lift your head and shoulders, reaching for your knees with your hands. Then lower back down very slowly.

- Begin this exercise gently and build up.

To ease back problems

- While feeding, always sit with your back well supported and straight. Use a pillow or cushion behind your waist.

- Kneel or squat to do low-level jobs like bathing your baby or picking things up off the floor. Avoid bending your back. Make your knees work instead. Change nappies on a waist-level surface or while kneeling on the floor.

- To lift weights like a carrycot or an older child, bend your knees, keep your back straight and hold the weight close to your body. Make your thigh muscles work as you lift.

- Try to keep a straight back when you push a pram or buggy, or carry your baby in a sling.

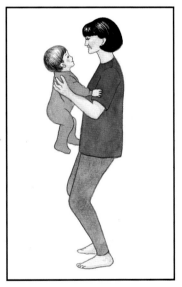

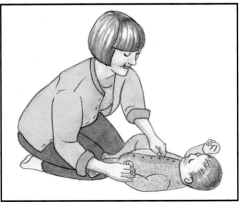

KEEPING HEALTHY

EATING

Being a parent is an exhausting business and it is easy to find that you have no time or energy to cook or eat properly. Try to make eating well a priority; it will make you feel better and needn't take lots of time. Have a look at the fast healthy foods shown on page 75 and try to follow the guidelines about eating a healthy diet explained on page 74.

If you are breastfeeding make sure you eat and drink plenty and don't go on a diet. The section on page 10 provides information about what to eat when breastfeeding.

If you're not breastfeeding and feel you need to lose weight, talk to your doctor about it first. Cut down on fat and sugar and don't go on a crash diet. Small regular meals will keep up your energy levels without adding to your weight.

PHYSICAL ACTIVITY

When you're feeling tired, being more active or taking more exercise may seem like the last thing you need. But activity can relax you, help your body recover after childbirth, keep you fit or improve your fitness, and makes you feel better.

- **Keep up the postnatal exercises you were taught.** Stick at them. They'll strengthen vital muscles and improve your shape. Some important exercises are described on page 114.

- **Join a postnatal exercise class if you've recently had a baby**. Company may help. Find out if your local maternity unit has a class run by an obstetric

'I think everyone assumes that after the first month or so, you're back to normal again. But I know from talking to friends that I'm not the only one to feel like anything but normal.'

'A frump. That's what I am. But where's the time to do anything about it.'

'I just don't like myself any more. My whole body's completely changed.'

'You think you're the only person in the world with this problem, and you feel embarrassed and, you know, almost a bit ashamed, as though somehow it's your fault. So you just get on and try to forget about it or hope it will go away. And when it doesn't, you get really fed up. It was only because I got talking to a friend, and we found out we both felt the same, it was only then that I started to think, well, maybe I can do something about this. And because there were two of us, we had a bit more courage and could back each other up.'

If you have a problem that is bothering you, don't ignore it – ask for help. Your doctor may be able to suggest treatment or might refer you to a specialist at the hospital or to an obstetric physiotherapist who can help with back and bladder problems and painful stitches.

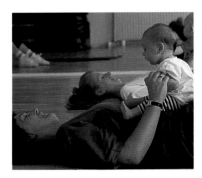

THREE GOOD REASONS TO STOP SMOKING

- *Your children's health will improve.*

- *Your health will improve.*

- *You'll have money to spend on other things.*

FOR HELP

Contact Quitline (see page 136). Their counsellors will give you help, advice or just encouragement. Their lines are open 24 hours a day and they can also give you details of your nearest quit smoking group. In Northern Ireland, contact the Ulster Cancer Foundation (see page 136). In Scotland, call Smokeline (see page 136). The Stop smoking made easier leaflet is available from the HEA.

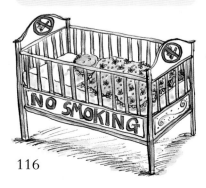

physiotherapist, or ask your health visitor about other local classes. If it isn't a special postnatal class be sure to tell the person running the class if you've had a baby in the last few months. You'll need to take special care of your back and avoid exercises that could damage it.

- **Push the pram or buggy briskly, remembering to keep your back straight**. Get out for walks as much as you can.

- **Play energetic games with older children**. Make yourself run about as well as them. Find outdoor space if there's no space at home.

- **Run upstairs**. You probably find yourself going up and down a hundred times a day in any case. Try to look on it as good exercise!

- **Squat down to pick things up from the floor holding heavy weights close to your body**. This is also something you're likely to be doing a lot. If you squat rather than stoop, bending your knees and keeping your back straight, you'll improve your thigh muscles. You'll also avoid damaging your back.

- **Join an exercise class**. There may be one locally that welcomes children or has a crèche. Ask your health visitor.

- **Swimming is good, relaxing exercise**. If you take your child with you, try to have someone else there too, so that you get a chance to swim.

- **Borrow or buy an exercise video**. Do a workout at home, perhaps with a friend. Get the children to join in.

QUIT SMOKING

Many people smoke because they believe that smoking calms their nerves, but it doesn't. It just calms the craving for nicotine that cigarettes create. So here are some useful steps to stop smoking.

- **Know why you want to stop**. It is handy to keep a checklist of your reasons to stop smoking.

- **Change your habits.** Smoking is strongly linked to some situations – the first cigarette of the day, the cigarette with tea or coffee, when the phone rings. Try to break the link by changing your habits. For example drink orange juice instead of coffee for a while.

- **Be ready to stop**. Choose a day and stop completely on that day. The day before get rid of cigarettes, ashtrays and lighters.

- **Get support.** Tell family and friends you have decided to stop and ask them for their support. For example ask them not to offer you a cigarette.

- **Anticipate problems**. Which situations will be difficult? Don't just wait for them to happen. Plan how to deal with them.

- **Take one day at a time.** At the beginning of each day, congratulate yourself on having made it so far, but make your goal to get through today without smoking. Never mind tomorrow.

- **If you need to put something in your mouth, try sugar-free chewing gum or something healthy, and non-fattening.** If you need to do something with your hands, find something to fiddle with – a pencil, coin – anything but a cigarette.

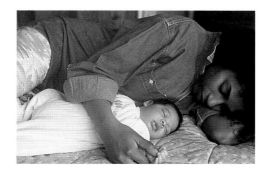

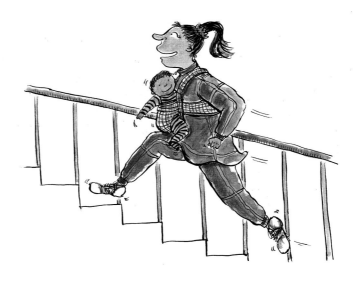

SLEEP

Most of the time parents just live with tiredness. But when the tiredness begins to make you feel low, bad-tempered, unable to cope and certainly unable to enjoy things, you've got to find ways of getting more sleep or at least more rest. Just one day, one night, one week, could help.

● **Get to bed early, really early, say for a week**. If you can't sleep when you get to bed, do something relaxing for half an hour beforehand, whether it's exercise, or soaking in a bath, or watching television.

● **Deep relaxation can refresh you after only five or ten minutes**. So it's worth learning a relaxation technique. You may find books, tapes or videos about this at your library.

● **Sleep when your baby sleeps**. Rest when (if) your child has a daytime rest, or is at playgroup or nursery school. Arrange for a relative or friend to take your child for a while, not so that you can get the jobs done, but so you can sleep. Take turns with other parents to give yourself time to rest. Set an alarm if you're worried about sleeping too long.

● **If you can, share getting up in the night with your partner**. Take alternate nights or weeks. If you're on your own, a friend or relative may be prepared to have your children overnight occasionally.

● **Look on page 56 for other ways of coping with disturbed nights**.

● **Do something about any stress**. Tiredness often comes from stress (see below). If you can do something about the stress, you may be able to cope better, even without more sleep.

COPING WITH STRESS

Small children ask a lot of you, and there's a limit to what you can ask of them. But perhaps the greatest stress comes from coping with the rest of life at the same time as coping with a baby or small child. You can spend a whole day trying to get one job done, but never managing to fit it in. Just as you start on it, your baby wakes up, or a nappy needs changing, or your child wants attention. Sometimes you can feel as though life is completely out of control. And if you're not the sort of person who can take things as they come and not mind about what is or isn't done, you can get to feel very tense and frustrated.

'I think the tiredness is the worst thing. It goes on and on. And you've got no choice, you've got to keep going. So you feel sort of trapped. And after a bit, it gets you down, feeling so tired all the time.'

'You come in from work and you start right in on another job. And then when you've got them off to bed, there are still other things you've got to do. So you drop into bed and there's been no breathing space. You're probably up in the night as well. And then you get up the next morning and start all over again.'

(A FATHER)

'It's the two of them. What one wants the other doesn't want. When I'm getting the little one off to sleep, the older one suddenly decides he needs the potty. You can't seem to do right by both of them. You're split in two, and there's no let-up, it's the whole time.'

117

'It's hard to explain to someone who isn't a parent how, even when you're enjoying it, there's this sort of constant drain on you. You think about them all the time, you have to. You have to think for them all the time. Even when I'm out at work, I have to think about getting back on time, and remembering to tell the childminder something, and buying something for tea …'

'It gets so frustrating. I wake up in the morning and think, "Right, what have I got today?" And then I give myself a great big long list of all the things I've got to do, and if I can't get them all done in that day, I get really narked about it.'

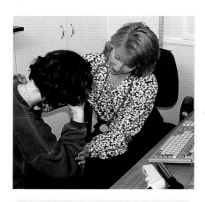

Alcohol may appear to help you relax and unwind. In fact it's a depressant, affecting moods, judgement, self-control, and co-ordination. If you're tired and run down, it affects these even more. So watch how much and when you drink. Never mix alcohol with anti-depressants or tranquillisers.

Stress also comes from worry and unhappiness: maybe to do with the place you live, money, relationships or just a lot of small, but important things. You may not be able to change the way your children are or the life you lead. But you may be able to do something about the stress. It's a matter of finding solutions that are right for you.

● You may find that you can relax just by doing something that you enjoy for half an hour in the evening when you can put other things out of your mind for a while. A bath, maybe, or time to look at a magazine or the television. Do whatever will wind you down. Borrow a book or tape from the library about relaxation. Make yourself do it.

● See other people – it does take the pressure off. Try a mother and baby or parent and toddler group. Ask your health visitor or other parents about local groups. Or, if you're not keen on organised groups, get together with people you meet at the clinic, playgroup or nursery school.

● Relationships can go wrong when you're tense and tired and never seem to see each other, so make time to be with your partner, even if only to fall asleep together in front of the television.

● Talking about the stress you're feeling can help to get rid of it, at least for a while. If you and your partner can understand how each other is feeling, then take time to talk about how best to support each other. Sometimes it's better to talk with people outside the family (see page 120).

● Make the very most of all the help you can find. And give up a bit. You can't do everything. Try

to believe it really doesn't matter.

● There are no prizes for being a supermum or superdad. Compromise if you're a perfectionist.

FEELING DEPRESSED

(see also **Postnatal depression** on page 6)

Most of us feel low occasionally and lack of sleep, stress, and may be the strain of balancing paid work and parenting, and money problems, all contribute to making the early stages of parenthood a difficult, as well as a rewarding, time. Sometimes feeling low takes over completely and becomes depression.

Depression is more than feeling unhappy. It's feeling hopeless about yourself and all that's happening to you. The hopelessness can make you angry. But often you feel too tired even for anger. It can seem as though there's no answer and no end to the way you're feeling. You may feel all, or some, of these things:

● tired, but can't sleep;
● no appetite or are overeating;
● no interest in yourself;
● no interest in your baby;
● the smallest chores are almost impossible to manage;
● you never stop crying.

This kind of depression is like an illness. Nothing seems worth doing, so doing anything as demanding as caring for a baby or child becomes a real struggle. Both for yourself and for the family, it's important to get help.

See your GP or health visitor, or both. Take someone with you if this would help. Make it clear that you're not talking about just feeling low but something more worrying than that. You may find that you're too low even to make the first step. If this is the case it's important to talk to someone – your partner, a friend or your mother, and ask them to talk to your GP or health visitor on your behalf and arrange an appointment for you.

Talking it through
It does help to talk, but it may be very hard to do so.

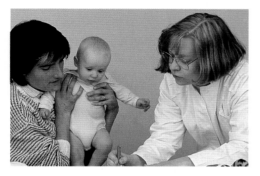

- You may want to say things that you're afraid of admitting to the people you love.

- You may feel guilty about your feelings.

- You may believe that you'll be judged as a bad mother for admitting to your feelings.

For all these reasons it's often best to talk to someone who isn't close to you, someone to whom you can be honest without being afraid of shocking them.
 You may find that it's enough to talk to your GP or health visitor, or they may be able to refer you to someone else. If you can talk about how you feel you'll almost certainly find that the things you fear are not as bad as you thought they were.

Medical treatment
If you're feeling totally lost in depression, your doctor may prescribe anti-depressant drugs. They may be enough to give you the lift you need to start coping again, and then to find a way out of your depression, though they can take time to work. Anti-depressants are *not* habit-forming. You

should not be concerned about them if they are prescribed for you by your GP. Tranquillisers may also be offered. They are different. They don't help depression and can be habit-forming, so they're best avoided.

RELATIONSHIPS

PARTNERSHIPS UNDER STRAIN

Relationships are often strained by parenthood, no matter what they were like before. Part of the problem is that you have so much less time to spend with each other than you did before the baby arrived and it's so much harder to get out together and enjoy the things you used to do.

- Your partner may feel left out.

- You may feel resentful at what you see as lack of support.

The really hard time, when children take up all your energy, doesn't last for ever. Try to make time for each other when you can and do little things to make each other feel cared for and included.

TIME TO LISTEN

Don't expect your partner, however close you were before the baby was born, to read your mind. Things are changing in both your lives and you have to talk about it. Your partner will not know what you want unless you say what it is and will not understand why you're resentful or angry unless you explain what's bothering you.

- Ask a friend or relation to babysit so that you can have time together – even if it's just for a walk together in the park.

'It felt like an invasion. All of a sudden, everything was revolving around the baby. For the first month or two I found it really hard. Now it's three of us and it couldn't ever be different, I couldn't imagine it back with just the two of us, but it was a very hard feeling, adjusting to the invasion of our privacy.'

'I think Dave thinks I've got an easy life, you know, just being at home all day. He thinks I can just suit myself and do what I want to do. I get very angry because there are days when I'd give anything to be walking out of the house like he does.'

'There's a lot of pressure, it's true. I think we've had to learn a lot, and learn it fast, about how to get on when there's so much to cope with. But then there's a lot we both enjoy, and more to share, really.'

GETTING HELP

If this is your first baby you may be feeling very lonely and left out of your old life. Your partner can't supply everything that you used to get from work and friends. You need other people in your life too for support, friendship, and a shoulder to cry on. See Loneliness page 122.

If you feel your relationship is in danger of breaking down, get help. RELATE (National Marriage Guidance) has local branches where you can talk to someone in confidence, either with your partner or alone.

Counselling is offered on all sorts of relationship difficulties: you don't have to be married to contact marriage guidance.
To find your local branch, look under RELATE or Marriage Guidance in your phone book, or write to the address on page 135.

'I couldn't think about it. My mind was on the baby. And it sounds bad, but all my feelings seemed to be taken up by the baby too. And that caused a lot of difficulty for a while. I did feel bad about it, as though it was my fault. But you can't make love as an obligation, can you? I mean, you can, but it's not really any good for either of you.'

(A FATHER)

- Share the housework to make more time just to be together.

- Share the babycare too.

- Talk about how you should bring up your children. You may find that you don't agree about basic matters such as discipline and attitudes. Try to work out a way of not always disagreeing in front of your children.

SEX

Babies and small children don't make for an easy sex life. Often you're tired, maybe too strained, and opportunities are limited. This hardly matters if both you and your partner are content. But if sex is a problem in any way at all, it's important to look at what you can do. Unhappy sex, or just lack of it, can cause a lot of frustration and worry and can really strain relationships.

Immediately after the baby is born many women feel sore as well as tired. They may also be worried about the state of their body or about getting pregnant again.

Men can face problems too. Tiredness apart, a father's sexual feelings will probably be much the same as before his baby's birth. But many men worry about what's right for their partner, are unsure what to do, and feel worried and frustrated.

- **If penetration hurts, say so**. It's not pleasant to have sex if it causes you pain and if you pretend everything is all right when it isn't you may well start seeing sex as a chore rather than a pleasure, which won't help either of you. You can still give each other pleasure without penetration.

- **Be careful the first few times**. Explore a bit with your own fingers first to reassure yourself that it won't hurt and use plenty of extra lubrication such as lubricating jelly: hormone changes after childbirth may

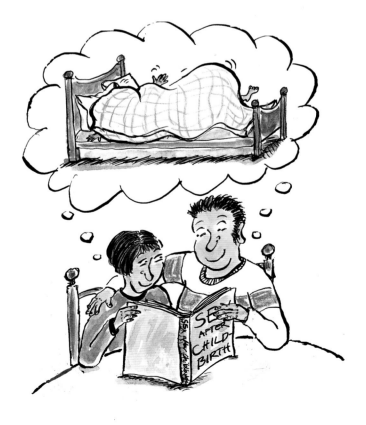

mean that you don't lubricate as much as usual.

- **Make time to relax together.** There's little point trying to make love when your minds are on anything but each other.

- **Sort out contraception.** It's possible to become pregnant again soon after the birth of a baby, even if you're breastfeeding, and even if you haven't started your period again. So if you don't want to conceive again quickly, you need to use some kind of contraception from the start. Contraception is usually discussed before you leave hospital after your child's birth, and at the postnatal check-up. But you can go at any time, before or after a check-up, to your GP or family planning clinic, or talk with your health visitor.

- **If your baby sleeps in the same room as you**, you may have to move either yourselves or your baby before you can relax enough to have sex.

- **Don't rush. Take time.**

- **If you're still experiencing pain two months or so after the birth, talk to your doctor or family planning clinic about it.** Treatment is available for a painful episiotomy scar. Ask to see an obstetric physiotherapist.

LONE PARENTS

Bringing a baby into your life changes your relationships with other people whether you're part of a couple or alone with your child.

Some lone mothers feel that their own mothers are taking over, others resent the fact that their mothers won't help them more.

However painful it may be, it's best to try to be very clear about the kind of help you do want, rather than going along with what's offered and then feeling resentful. Remember your mother is also having to get used to a completely new relationship with you and she won't know what to do for the best – unless you tell her!

You may find that your old friends stop coming by or that they seem to expect you just to drop everything and go out for the evening. Try not to get angry with them. They don't understand the changes you are going through. Keep in touch and keep some space for them in your life. Friends can be more valuable than money when the going gets tough.

You may be amazed and delighted at how much help you'll get from relations and friends if you ask! But the best support will probably come from other lone mothers.

- Suggest a 'swap' arrangement with another parent so that you take it in turns to look after both the children, by day to begin with, and later overnight. The children will benefit too from having a close friend, especially if they've no brothers and sisters.

- Suggest a regular evening babysit by a trusted relation or friend. You may well find that they're delighted at the opportunity of making friends with your child.

- Grandparents are often glad to have a baby overnight, even if they don't much care for babysitting.

'It's not talked about, is it? Except as a sort of joke. So you don't know if you've got a problem or not. At first, Paula found it hurt, and it put us both off and frightened us a bit. We were worried because we didn't know whether that was normal.'

(A FATHER)

'The thing is everything's on your shoulders. When you have to decide something, you know, like whether or not to take him to the doctor, or even everyday small things, there's nobody to share that with. There are so many things it's useful to talk about, and if you're on your own, you can't. If there's a crisis, you're on your own.'

'It's less stressful being your own boss. There's more satisfaction somehow, more achievement. There's no one to disagree with, no conflict over discipline, no competition with other adults.'

'There's no company in the evenings. That's almost the hardest part. You put the kids to bed at night and that's it.'

121

'At home in Pakistan, there's a lot of visiting, lots of people about, and children can go anywhere. Here there isn't so much coming and going. You can feel very isolated.'

'When I was working, there were lots of people to talk to and I had all the company I needed. Now I haven't got any of that, I really miss it. And I think I've lost confidence. I don't find it so easy to talk to people.'

'We first met at a postnatal group which the health visitor organised. We were all really shy at first, but after six weeks of meeting we all wanted to meet again, so we swapped addresses and agreed to meet on Tuesday mornings. That was three years ago. We have had our second babies now and our older ones are great friends – they go to nursery together and stay over at each other's houses. That postnatal group was the best thing that ever happened to me!'

YOUR FEELINGS

You'll almost certainly want (and need) to talk about your own feelings. Try to find another adult to talk to. Your children don't need to hear the details of your feelings about their father and will feel confused and unhappy about loving someone who you clearly do not love.

MAKING NEW FRIENDS

If you don't already know people locally, try contacting other, mothers through local groups.

- Ask your health visitor what's going on locally, and look through the list of support and information organisations on pages 133–6. Many run local groups.

- Gingerbread, a self-help organisation run by and for one-parent families (address on page 135) has local groups around the country. Through these groups you can meet parents in similar situations to your own. And you can often help each other out as well as support each other generally.

MONEY AND HOUSING

Money may be a major headache. Look at **Rights and benefits** (pages 127-32) to check you're claiming all you're entitled to.

The National Council for One Parent Families (address on page 136) offers free advice packs to lone parents and will provide independent advice about maintenance problems to women on benefits.

If you need help with claiming maintenance contact the Child Support Agency helpline on 0345 139896 (local call charge). If you're on benefits your case will be handled automatically. If you're not on benefits, and want the agency to assess and collect maintenance on your behalf, there is a fee.

See page 125 for information about help with housing problems. If you are working, or thinking of it, see page 132 for information about help with getting back to work.

ABSENT FATHERS

If you'd hoped to bring up your child as a couple you may be feeling very angry and hurt. One of the hardest things for a lone mother is to keep her hurt, angry feelings to herself and let her child make a different relationship with his or her father.

Unless your child's father is violent to you or the child, or you feel he's likely to abuse the child in some way, it's almost certainly better for your child's own development if he or she is able to see his or her father regularly, even if you remarry.

You may find that your child behaves badly at first when he or she gets home. Small children aren't able to understand and explain how they're feeling and this is the only way they have of letting you know that they're confused. Unless you're convinced that something bad is happening on access visits, the best thing is to be reassuring and calm. In the end your child will learn to look forward to visits and also to coming home.

LONELINESS

Lots of mothers feel lonely. Especially after the birth of a first baby, many find that they're cut off from old friends, but it's difficult to make new ones. Getting out to see people, even if you've got people to see, is often an effort. Meeting new people takes confidence, but it's worth it. Having other people with whom to share the ups and downs of being a parent will help you to cope with the difficult times and make the good times better.

- Ask your health visitor for information about postnatal groups, mother and baby groups, parent and toddler groups, and playgroups. These may be advertised on the clinic notice board.

- Chat with other mothers at your baby or child health clinic.

- Talk to your health visitor and ask for an introduction to other new mothers living nearby.

- MAMA, HomeStart, the National Childbirth Trust, and many other local organisations, sometimes based in a church or temple, run local groups where you can meet other people, chat, relax and get a lot of support.

GOING BACK TO WORK

Most mothers go back to work at some point. About half do so before their children start school. It may help to talk to other working mothers. But also try to decide what's right for you and your family. (For information about childcare, see pages 47–50.) You'll need to think about the following.

- **Feeding** – If your baby is still breastfeeding, try to get him or her used to taking milk from a bottle or cup before you return to work. If you need help with combining work and feeding, discuss it with your health visitor, the National Childbirth Trust, La Leche League, or the Association for Breastfeeding Mothers (see page 133). You can express milk to leave for feeds. It's also possible to give your baby formula milk in the middle of the day and still breastfeed the rest of the time.

- **Childcare arrangements** – must be as simple as possible to work smoothly. If they don't work

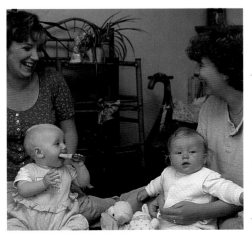

smoothly, there's a lot of strain. You also have to be reasonably sure they'll go on working over time.

- **Paying for childcare**. – can you afford to pay for childcare out of what you earn? Can you find work that you can do while your partner is at home? Can you fit work into school hours? Can a relation help out? Is there any subsidised childcare in your area? (See page 124.)

- **Housework** – when and who'll do it? If you have a partner you need to talk about how you'll divide responsibilities for housework and childcare.

- **Making time for your child** – even the best childcare isn't a substitute for a parent. Children need to know that they're special. If you work long hours during the week, can you or your partner keep your weekends completely free? If you don't see your child in the day, can you keep him or her up late in the evening and compensate with long daytime sleeps? You may be able to work flexi-time, part-time, or a four-day week, and make a special time to be with your child.

'At first I hated leaving her. It was much more upsetting than I'd thought – but more for me than for her, really. I'm better about it now, especially as time goes by and I can see that she's happy and well looked after and I've got to know and like the person who cares for her. But I don't think you can ever feel completely right about it. So you just have to live with that and get on with it.'

'There's no doubt it's hard work. I mean, there's no evenings off, because it's then that we have to get all the jobs done round the house. To my mind, families where there's one parent at home all the time have it very easy in comparison.'

'I enjoy the job. It's nothing much, but it earns money we need, and it gets me out and makes me do things I'd not do otherwise. I think I'm a better parent for doing it. I like having contact with people other than mothers. And Darren gets to meet other children, and he thrives on that.'

*Some mothers find the answer to feeling lonely and cut off is to take a job. It's not always easy to find the right sort of work with the right sort of hours, or to make childcare arrangements. But if you feel that work outside the home could help, read the **Going back to work** section.*

123

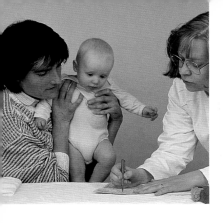

8 Your services

There are a wide range of services available from statutory organisations, voluntary organisations and local groups. This chapter will help you find what you need. (Additional information for those living in Scotland and Northern Ireland can be found on page 126)

HEALTH SERVICES

COMMUNITY MIDWIVES

Your community midwife has a legal duty to care for you and your baby for the first ten days after your baby's birth and will keep you on her books for the first 28 days if you, or the baby, need her. She can help with any problem to do with you or your baby and will give you a phone number to call at any time, day or night, if you need to.

HEALTH VISITORS

Your health visitor usually makes her first visit some time after your baby is ten days old. After that she may only see you at clinics or when you ask to see her. If you're alone, or struggling, she may make a point of coming by to see whether you need any help.

A health visitor is a qualified nurse who has had extra training to become a health visitor. Part of her role is to help families, especially families with babies and young children, to avoid illness and keep healthy. Talk to your health visitor if you feel anxious, depressed or worried about your children. She may be able to offer advice and suggest where to find help, and may organise groups where you can meet other mothers.

Your health visitor can visit you at home, or you can see her at your child health clinic, doctor's surgery or health centre, depending on where she's based. She'll give you a phone number to get in touch if you need to.

FAMILY DOCTORS

Your family doctor (GP) can be contacted at any time for yourself, your baby, or child. Some doctors will see small babies at the beginning of surgery hours or without an appointment if necessary, but be prepared to wait. Some will give advice over the phone. Most doctors provide developmental reviews and immunisation themselves, or you can go to a child health clinic.

CHILD HEALTH CLINICS

Your child health clinic offers regular health and development reviews (see page 36) and immunisation (see pages 94-101) for your baby or child. It's run by health visitors and doctors. You can talk about any problems to do with your child, but if your child is ill and is likely to need treatment, you should go to your GP.

At some child health clinics you can get baby milk and vitamins cheaper than in the shops. If you're entitled to free baby milk and vitamins, or to low price baby milk, you may be able to get these at your clinic. Clinics are good places to meet other parents. Some run mother and baby or parent and toddler groups, and sell secondhand baby clothes and equipment.

COMMUNITY HEALTH COUNCILS

Your community health council (CHC; in your phone book under the name of your health authority) can advise you on how to get what you need from the health services and on what you're entitled to. It can also give you information about local services. For example, if you want to change your doctor, your CHC will have a list of local doctors and may know something about them.

LOCAL AUTHORITY SERVICES

SOCIAL SERVICES DEPARTMENTS

Your social services department (in your phone book under the name of your local authority) can give you information about most services for parents and children – day nurseries, childminders, playgroups, opportunity groups (which

REGISTER YOUR BABY WITH YOUR DOCTOR

Register your baby with your doctor as early as possible with the pink card (yellow card in Northern Ireland) that you'll be given when you register your baby's birth at the local registry office. Sign the card and take or send it to your doctor. If you need the doctor to see your baby before you've registered the birth, you can go to the surgery and fill in a registration form for the doctor there.

If you move, register with a new doctor close to you as soon as possible (see page 125).

include children with special needs), family centres, and so on. Many local authorities produce booklets listing local services for families with under-fives. Ask at your local library, social services department, citizens' advice bureau or other advice centre.

SOCIAL WORKERS

Social workers are usually in social services departments. Their job is to provide support for people in need in their area who are having difficulty coping, financially or practically. A social worker may be able to get your child a nursery place, help you find better housing, or give you information about your rights.

To contact a social worker, phone your local social services department. Or ask your health visitor to put you in touch.

HOUSING DEPARTMENTS

The housing department (in your phone book under the name of your local authority) is responsible for all council housing in your area and will run the council housing waiting list.

The housing department has a legal duty to house people in certain priority groups who are homeless (or are soon going to be) through no fault of their own. Priority groups include pregnant women and parents of children under 16.

Through your housing department you should also be able to find out about local housing associations, which also provide housing for rent.

EDUCATION DEPARTMENTS

Your education department (in your phone book under the name of your local authority) is responsible for all the state-run nursery schools, nursery classes and infant schools in your area and can give you information about them.

The education department also has a responsibility to assess children with special needs and provide suitable education for them.

ADVICE CENTRES

Advice centres are any non-profit making agencies that give advice on benefits, housing and other problems. They include citizens' advice bureaux, community law centres, welfare rights offices, housing aid centres, neighbourhood centres and community projects. Look for them under these names in your phone book, or under the name of your local authority.

USING THE SERVICES

If you're to get the best from these services it helps to be clear about what you want.

- Before you meet with any professional, think through exactly what you want to talk about and what information you can give that'll be helpful. You may want to make some notes beforehand and take them with you as a reminder.

- Unless your child needs to be with you, try to get a friend or neighbour to look after him or her so that you can concentrate. It's much easier to talk and listen if you're not distracted.

- If you do have to go with your child or children, take books or toys with you to entertain them.

- Try to consider the answers or advice given to you. If your immediate feeling is 'but that wouldn't work for me' or 'that isn't what I'm looking for', then say so and try to talk about it. You're less likely to come away with an answer you're not happy with or can't put into practice.

- If a problem is making life difficult or is really worrying you, it's worth keeping going until you get some kind of answer, if not a solution. So if the first person you talk to can't help, ask if they can suggest where else you might go. Or if the doctor or health visitor suggests a remedy that doesn't work, go back and ask again.

- Some professionals aren't good at explaining things. If you don't understand, then say so. It's their responsibility to be clear, not yours to guess what they meant. Go back over what's said to you to get it straight.

- If your first language is not English, you may be able to get the help of a linkworker or health advocate. Their job is not just to translate the words, but to act as a friend and make sure that the professionals understand just what you need. Ask your health visitor if there's a linkworker or health advocate in your area.

HOW TO CHANGE YOUR GP

You may need to change your GP if you move. You

125

'I think looking after children is the hardest job going and the one you get least preparation for.'

SCOTLAND AND NORTHERN IRELAND

Community health councils
In Scotland, community health councils are called Local Health Councils. In Northern Ireland they are called Health and Social Services Councils. Look in your phone book under the name of your local health board, or local Health and Social Services Board.

Social services departments
In Scotland, the social services department is called the Social Work Department (in your phone book under the name of your local regional council). In Northern Ireland, look in your phone book under your local Health and Social Services Board.

Housing departments
In Scotland, you will find your housing department in your phone book under the name of your local district council. In Northern Ireland, the housing department is called the Northern Ireland Housing Executive (in your phone book under Housing Executive).

Education departments
In Scotland, you will find your education department in your phone book under the name of your local regional council. In Northern Ireland, the education department is called the Education and Library Board (in your phone book under Education and Library Board).
Note: In this publication, the NHS also refers to the Northern Ireland Health and Personal Social Services.

may want to change for other reasons, even if you're not moving house.

First find a GP who will accept you. See if anybody can recommend one. Your local community health council (CHC) or health authority (in Scotland your local health board; in Northern Ireland your local Health and Social Services Board; the Central Services Agency in Belfast) keeps a list of doctors in your area. You may have to try more than one GP before you find one willing to accept you, especially if you live in a heavily populated area. If you can't find someone after several attempts, your health authority will do it for you and should send them your medical card if you have it, or the address of your previous GP if not. When you call at the surgery of the GP you've chosen, you may be asked why you want to change. You don't have to give a reason but if you do, try to avoid criticising your old GP. Say something good about the new one instead. For example, the surgery may be easier to get to, the hours may be better, the GP may have a good reputation for treating young children, the practice may be larger and provide more, or you may prefer a woman doctor, or one who shares your cultural background.

Once you've found a GP to accept you, leave your medical card with the receptionist. You don't have to contact your old GP at all. If you've lost your medical card, your new GP will probably ask you to complete a form instead, although sometimes you may be asked to contact the health authority (in the phone book under the name of your health authority) giving the name and address of your previous GP, to obtain a

medical card first. If you don't know your old GP's name and address this may take a while, but if you need treatment in the meantime, you can approach any GP, who must take you on, at least temporarily. It's best to say from the beginning that you need treatment now if you're also asking to be permanently registered with that GP.

FINDING OTHER HELP
The help you want may not best come from the services of professionals. There are many other sources of help available to parents – not only family and friends, but also many different kinds of local groups and voluntary organisations.

LOCAL GROUPS
To find out about local groups:

- Ask your health visitor or GP.

- Ask at your citizens' advice bureau or other advice centre, your local library, your social services department, or your local Council for Voluntary Service (in your phone book, maybe as Voluntary Action Group, Rural Community Council or Volunteer Bureau). (In Northern Ireland, contact the Northern Ireland Council for Voluntary Action. In Scotland, contact the Scottish Council for Voluntary Organisations.)

- Look on notice-boards in your child health clinic, health centre, GP's waiting room, local library, advice centres, supermarket, newsagent or toy shop.

- Look through the list of national organisations (pages 133-136). Many run local groups.

In many areas there are now groups offering support to parents who share the same background and culture. Many of these are women's or mothers' groups. Your health visitor may know if there's such a group in your area. Or ask at places like your local library, your citizens' advice bureau or other advice or community centre, your local Council for Voluntary Service, or your Community Relations Council (in your phone book, maybe as Council for Racial Equality or Community Relations Office).

STARTING A GROUP
If you can't find a local group that suits you or can't find the support you need, think about setting it up for yourself. Many local groups have begun through a couple of mothers (say with crying babies, or sleepless toddlers, or just fed up and lonely) getting together and talking. You could advertise on your clinic notice-board or in a newsagent's window or local newspaper. Or ask your health visitor to put you in touch with others in the same situation as yourself. You don't have to offer any more than a place to meet and a few cups of coffee. Or you could get a copy of New Lives (direct from the Maternity Alliance, price £3.00 see page 136), which has suggestions for how to set up a new mothers' group.

9 Your rights and benefits

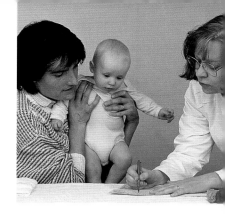

The following pages are a guide to the main benefits available to families with young children. You may qualify for other benefits too. It's always worth checking that you're claiming everything to which you are entitled. The figures given are accurate up to March 1998.

WHERE TO GET ADVICE AND HELP

Working out what benefits you're entitled to and making claims can be complicated. Get help if you need it.

- You can go to your social security office (in the phone book under 'Benefits Agency'; in Northern Ireland under 'Social Security Agency'). Or go to your local citizen's advice bureau or other advice centre (see page 135); or, in Northern Ireland, to the Benefit Shop, Castle Court, Royal Avenue, Belfast. Many social security offices are very busy and an advice centre is often the best place to go.
- Some local authorities have welfare rights officers. Phone your social services depart- ment (in Scotland, social work department, in Northern Ireland, Health and Social Services Board) and ask.
- Some voluntary organisations offer information and advice on benefits. See page 135 for details.

Rates of benefits are not given here as they change every year, but you can find them in leaflet NI196 (in Northern Ireland, NIL96), Social security benefit rates.

FOR PARENTS

CHILD BENEFIT

This is a tax-free weekly payment made to almost anybody responsible for a child under 16. You can also claim for a child aged between 16 and 19 who's in full-time education not above A-level or an equivalent standard. In addition, Child Benefit may be extended for a few weeks for school leavers aged 16 and 17 who register for work or youth training. (In Northern Ireland, register at an office of the Department of Economic Development.) Child Benefit is not means-tested. You get a higher rate for the first child than for other children.

Child Benefit is paid:

- for each child you are responsible for (you don't have to be the parent to claim); every four weeks by a payment card or book of orders which you cash at the post office, or direct into most banks or building society accounts. If you are a one-parent family or on Family Credit, income-based Jobseeker's Allowance or Income Support (see page 130, you can choose to be paid weekly.

LEAFLETS GIVING GENERAL INFORMATION

- *FB8 Babies and benefits. A guide to benefits for expectant and new mothers.*
- *FB27 Bringing up children? A guide to benefits for families with children.*
- *FB28 Sick or disabled? A guide to benefits if you're sick or disabled for a few days or more.*
- *FB2 Which benefit? A short guide to all social security benefits.*
- *NI 196 Social security benefit rates*

Government leaflets giving more information about particular benefits are listed under each benefit. You can get these leaflets from: your local social security office some large post offices your citizens advice bureau or other advice centre

HOW TO CLAIM

You may receive a Child Benefit claim pack automatically. If you do not, then you can get one from your social security office or post office. Or you can use the form on the back of the leaflet FB8 Babies and benefits which you can get from post offices and clinics.

You need to send your baby's birth certificate (see page 130). It will be returned to you. If you claim late you can be paid in arrears for up to 3 months.

If you're a couple (married or unmarried) the child's mother should claim. If a couple separates and lives with other partners one of the child's natural parents should claim.

If you are bringing up the child on your own (you're not living with anyone as husband and wife), you get a special higher rate of child benefit but only for the first child. Before April 1997 this was called One Parent Benefit. You won't get it if you're getting other benefits such as Widowed Mother's Allowance or Invalid Care Allowance for the same child.

FOR PREGNANT WOMEN

MATERNITY LEAVE

Every woman who is employed while she is pregnant is entitled to 14 weeks maternity leave. This right applies to every employee who gives the required notice (see below). If you have worked for the same employer for two years by the end of the 12th week before your baby is due, you will qualify for extended maternity absence which is up to 29 weeks from the week of childbirth.

To get maternity leave, you must write to your employer at least 21 days before you start your leave telling them:

- that you are pregnant
- the expected week of childbirth.
- the date you intend to start your maternity leave, but you only need to put this in writing if your employer asks for it.

If requested, you must also enclose your maternity certificate (form MAT B1; in Northern Ireland, form MB1) which your midwife or GP will give to you when you are about six months pregnant. If you can't give 21 days' notice, for example, if you have to go into hospital unexpectedly, you must write to your employer as soon as you reasonably can.

If you qualify for extended maternity absence you must give the same notice as above and at the same time you must inform

your employer in writing that you intend to return to work after the birth of your baby.

For more information about your maternity rights ask at the Jobcentre for the booklet PL958 Maternity Rights or send a stamped self-addressed envelope enclosing an extra first class stamp to The Maternity Alliance (see page 136) and ask for the leaflet Pregnant at Work.

STATUTORY MATERNITY PAY (SMP)

This is a payment for pregnant women inemployment. You can get it if:

- you've worked for the same employer for at least 26 weeks by the 15th week before the week your baby is due (this is called the 'qualifying week'). To work out which is the qualifying week, look on the calendar for the Sunday before (or on) which your baby is due. Not counting that Sunday, count back 15 Sundays. The qualifying week begins on that Sunday. See the example on the calendar here.
- your average weekly earnings are £62 or more during the eight weeks, (if you're paid weekly), or two months, (if you're paid monthly) before the end of the qualifying week. This period is approximately the 19th to 26th week of your pregnancy.

SMP payments

- SMP is paid for up to 18 weeks. For the first six weeks you get 90 % of your average pay, followed by 12 weeks at

the lower rate of SMP.

- SMP is paid by your employer, either weekly or monthly, depending on how you're normally paid. Tax and National Insurance contributions may be deducted.
- You can choose when to start getting your SMP. The earliest you can start getting your SMP is 11 weeks before the week the baby is due, but you can work right up to the birth without losing any of your SMP.
- SMP is paid even if you don't plan to return to work after your baby is born. You do not have to repay SMP if you don't return to work.
- SMP is only paid for weeks when you don't work. So if you only qualify for 14 weeks maternity leave then you will lose the last 4 of your 18 weeks of SMP when you go back to work.

How to claim

Write to your employer at least 21 days before you intend to stop work because of your pregnancy. Enclose your maternity certificate (form MAT B1; in Northern Ireland, form MB1), which is given to you by your doctor or midwife when you are about 26 weeks pregnant. If you don't get your maternity certificate in time, write to your employer anyway and send the form later. You may lose your right to SMP if you don't give 21 days' notice.

If you're unsure whether you can get SMP, ask your employer anyway. If you can't get SMP you may be able to claim Maternity

Allowance (see below).

MATERNITY ALLOWANCE

This is a benefit for pregnant women who've recently given up a job, or who are self-employed, or who are employed, but don't qualify for Statutory Maternity Pay (SMP).

You can claim it if you're not entitled to SMP (see above) but have worked and paid standard rate National Insurance contributions for at least 26 of the 66 weeks ending in the week before your baby is due.

Maternity Allowance payments

- There are two rates of Maternity Allowance. If you are self-employed or unemployed in the qualifying week (the 15th week before the expected week of childbirth), you get the lower rate. If you are employed in the qualifying week you get the higher rate.
- Maternity Allowance is paid for up to 18 weeks in the same way as SMP (see above). Payments start no earlier than 11 weeks before the week your baby is due.
- Payments are made only for the weeks when you're not working.
- It's paid directly into your bank or building society account or at your post office by a book of orders or a payment card.

How to claim

Send to your social security office (in Northern Ireland, Central Benefits Branch) the following:

A completed form MA1 (which you can get from your antenatal clinic or your social security office)
Your maternity certificate

(form MAT B1; in Northern Ireland, form MB1), which your doctor or midwife will give you when you are about 26 weeks pregnant. If you're claiming Maternity Allowance because you have been refused SMP, get form SMP1 from your employer and send this with your claim.

Claim as early as possible after you are 26 weeks pregnant. If you have not paid 26 weeks National Insurance contributions by this time, then you may decide to work later into your pregnancy; and you should send off form MA1 as soon as you have made 26 National Insurance contributions. You may lose benefit if you claim after the birth.

If you've worked in the last couple of years and paid National Insurance contributions, it's worth claiming Maternity Allowance even if you don't appear to qualify for it. You may be able to get some Incapacity Benefit if you've paid enough National Insurance contributions in earlier tax years. If you claim Maternity Allowance, but don't qualify for it, you should automatically be considered for Incapacity Benefit (you don't have to apply on a different form). Incapacity Benefit is paid from the 6th week before the baby is due until two weeks after the baby is born.

OTHER BENEFITS

When pregnant, and for a year after your baby is born, you will qualify for the following benefits.

LEAFLETS
*FB8 Babies and benefits
NI17A Maternity benefits
(in Northern Ireland,
NIL17A)*

● Free NHS prescriptions. To claim, ask your GP or midwife for form FW8 as soon as you're sure that you're pregnant and send it to your Health Authority (Health Board, in Scotland; or Central Services Agency in Northern Ireland).

● Free NHS dental treatment. To claim, simply tell your dentist that you're pregnant or have a baby under one year old.

● You may be able to get a Maternity Payment from the Social Fund (see page 131).

● If you're on Income Support or income-based Jobseekers' Allowance (see page 130), you can get free milk and vitamins while you're pregnant or have a child under five. See page 131 for how to claim.

FOR FAMILIES
FAMILY CREDIT

This is a tax-free benefit for working families with children. It's not a loan and doesn't have to be paid back. To be able to get Family Credit you, or your partner, must be working at least 16 hours a week and you must have at least one child under 16 (or under 19 in full-time education up to or including A-level, or an equivalent standard).

You can qualify for Family Credit whether you're employed or self-employed, or whether you're a two-parent or one-parent family. You may be single, married, or living with a partner as if you were married. Your right to Family Credit, and how much you get, depends on your and your partner's net income, how many children you have and what age they are, and what savings you and your partner have. If you or your partner work for more than 30 hours a week you can earn more

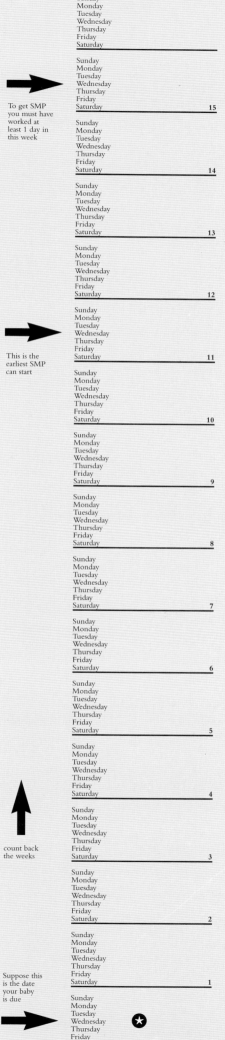

To get SMP you must have worked at least 1 day in this week   15

This is the earliest SMP can start   11

count back the weeks

Suppose this is the date your baby is due   1

and still get Family Credit. If you pay for registered childcare you may be able to earn even more and still get Family Credit. You will not get Family Credit if you have more than £8,000 in savings.

Family Credit payments

● Family Credit is normally paid for 26 weeks at a time. In each 26-week period, the amount you get stays the same even if your earnings or other circumstances change during that time.
● It is normally paid every four weeks directly into your bank and building society account, or weekly at the post office by order book or payment card.

How to claim

Use the Family Credit claim pack FC1. Fill in the claim form and send to the Family Credit Unit (or, in Northern Ireland, the Family Credit Branch) in the envelope provided. There is a Family Credit Helpline on 01253 50 00 50.

Other benefits if you get Family Credit

● Free NHS prescriptions. Free NHS dental treatment.
● Free NHS sight tests and vouchers for glasses.
● Free travel to hospital for NHS treatment.
● You may qualify for Housing Benefit and Council Tax Benefit (see pages 130–131)
● You may also be able to get payments from the Social Fund (see page 131). For example, a Maternity Payment to help buy new things for your baby. If you've a child under one year old who's not being breastfed, you can buy dried baby milk at a reduced price. Take your Family Credit order book, or notice of award of

LEAFLETS
FC1 Family Credit claim pack HC11 Help with NHS costs WMV1 Welfare milk and vitamins

benefit, to your local maternity or child health clinic or welfare food distribution centre, to prove that you're getting Family Credit. You may also have to prove your baby's age by showing the birth certificate or child benefit order book.

INCOME-BASED JOBSEEKER'S ALLOWANCE (JSA) AND INCOME SUPPORT (IS)

These are benefits for people who do not have enough money to live on.
You can claim JSA: If you are over 18, and unemployed or working for less than 16 hours a week, and you are actively seeking work. If you are 16 or 17 years old you can claim JSA if you have a child (but if you're single it's better to claim IS), or earlier if you face severe hardship.
You can claim IS: If you are over 16 and you are unemployed or work less than 16 hours a week and you do not have to be available for work because: either you're a lone parent, or you're pregnant and incapable of work, or you're pregnant and within the period of 11 weeks before the baby is due until 7 weeks after the baby is born, or you're disabled, or you're sick. You cannot claim JSA or IS if you have a partner who works for more than 24 hours a week or if you have savings of more than £8,000. How much you get depends on your age, the size of your family, your income, and other benefits you are getting (such as Child Benefit). The amount will be reduced if you have savings over £3,000. If you're

earning or claiming other benefits, your income will be 'topped up' to the JSA/IS level for your family size.

How to claim

Claim JSA by going to the Jobcentre in person (postal applications are allowed if you live too far from the Jobcentre). Claim IS by writing to your social security office or fill in the coupon in leaflet IS1 Income Support, which you can get from your social security office or post office. Your social security office will send a detailed postal claim for you to complete.

Other benefits if you get income-based Jobseeker's Allowance or Income Support

● Housing Benefit if you pay rent; and, in Northern Ireland, also if you pay rates (see Housing).
● Council Tax Benefit (see page 131); this does not apply in Northern Ireland.
● Free NHS prescriptions.
● Free NHS dental treatment.
● Free NHS sight tests and vouchers for glasses.
● Free travel to hospital for NHS treatment.
● You can get tokens for one free pint of milk a day for yourself while you are pregnant or breastfeeding and for each child under the age of five. If your baby is under one-year-old and you are bottlefeeding, you can exchange the tokens for dried baby milk at a maternity or child health clinic or a welfare food distribution centre.

How to claim

If you or someone in your family becomes pregnant, you should tell the social security office and let them

know the date the baby is due. Show them proof from the doctor or midwife. If you collect your benefit from the post office you can collect your milk tokens at the same time, or they will be posted to you if your benefit is paid directly into your bank account.

● You can also get free vitamins for yourself while you're pregnant or breastfeeding, and for any children under the age of five. You get them from a maternity or child health clinic or from a welfare food distribution centre. You do not need tokens but you may need to show proof that you are entitled (your benefit order book or notice of award of benefit) and proof of your children's ages (the birth certificate or child benefit order book).
● You may also be able to get payments from the Social Fund (see page 131). For example, a Maternity Payment to help buy new things for a baby.

HOUSING

Housing Benefit will help you pay your rent (and/or rates in Northern Ireland) if you're on income-based Jobseeker's Allowance, Income Support, or a low income. It will be paid direct to the council if you're a council tenant, or to you or your landlord if you're a private tenant.
How much you get depends on your income, savings, other benefits and family size. It may not be the same amount as the rent you are actually paying. You can't get Housing Benefit if you have savings of more than £16,000 and your benefit will be reduced if you have more than £3,000 in savings. If you've got a mortgage and

LEAFLETS
- F1S1 Income support
- IS20 A guide to Income Support
- JSAL5 Jobseeker's Allowance - Helping you back to work
- HC11 Help with NHS costs
- WMV 1 Welfare milk and vitamins

you're on income-based Jobseeker's Allowance or Income Support, you may be able to get help with your mortgage interest payments. See leaflet IS8 Help with housing costs (available from social security offices) for details.

How to claim

If you're getting Jobseeker's Allowance or Income Support you will get a Housing Benefit claim form with your JSA/IS claim form. Otherwise get a form from your local council. In Northern Ireland get the form from your Northern Ireland Housing Executive district office (for tenants) or the Rate Collection Agency local office (if you own your own home).

COUNCIL TAX BENEFIT

(not applicable in Northern Ireland) This benefit helps people on income-based Jobseeker's Allowance, Income Support, Family Credit or on a low income to pay their Council Tax. You can't get Council Tax Benefit if your savings are more than £16,000.

Most people on income-based Jobseeker's Allowance or Income Support can get 100 per cent of their Council Tax paid in benefit. For other low income families, how much benefit you get depends on your income and savings, and whether other adults live with you.

How to claim

If you're getting income-based Jobseeker's Allowance or Income Support you will get a Council Tax claim form with your JSA/IS claim form. Otherwise get a form from your local council.

HELP WITH NATIONAL HEALTH SERVICE COSTS

NHS BENEFITS FOR ALL CHILDREN UNDER 16

- Free NHS prescriptions.
- Free NHS dental treatment.
- Free NHS sight tests and vouchers for glasses.

YOUNG PEOPLE UNDER 19 AND STILL IN FULL-TIME EDUCATION

Young people under 19 and still in full-time education get free prescriptions, free dental treatment, free sight tests and vouchers for glasses. Those over 16, but not in full-time education get free dental treatment until they are 18.

NHS BENEFITS FOR ALL PREGNANT WOMEN AND MOTHERS OF BABIES UNDER ONE YEAR OLD

- Free NHS prescriptions.
- Free NHS dental treatment.

For how to claim see For pregnant women page 129.

NHS BENEFITS IF YOU GET FAMILY-CREDIT, INCOME-BASED JOBSEEKER'S ALLOWANCE OR INCOME SUPPORT

- Free NHS prescriptions.
- Free NHS dental treatment.
- Free NHS sight tests and vouchers for glasses.
- Free travel to hospital for NHS treatment.

- If you get income-based Jobseeker's Allowance or Income Support and are pregnant, breastfeeding or have a child under five, you can get tokens for free milk. You can also get free vitamins for yourself and your child. (Look under 'income-based Jobseeker's Allowance and Income Support' page 130 for how to claim.)
- If you get Family Credit and have a child under one year old, you can get dried baby milk at a reduced price (look under Family Credit page 129 for how to claim).

IF YOU DON'T GET FAMILY CREDIT OR INCOME- BASED JOBSEEKER'S ALLOWANCE OR INCOME SUPPORT BUT YOUR INCOME IS LOW

You may still get some help with NHS costs. Apply on form HC11 (which you can get from hospitals, dentists, and opticians as well as social security offices). Send it to the Health Benefits Division in the pre-paid envelope provided with the form. (In Northern Ireland you should send it to your social security office.) They will check your circumstances. If you qualify for help, you'll be sent a certificate of entitlement, setting out the amount of help you can get for each type of charge. The certificate is valid for six months.

If your circumstances change, write to the Health Benefits Division (or, in Northern Ireland, to your local social security office). They'll issue a fresh certificate if necessary.

THE SOCIAL FUND

The Social Fund offers help with certain expenses that are

LEAFLETS
- HC11 Help with NHS costs
- FB28 Sick or disabled?

difficult to meet out of your regular income.

- If you or your partner are getting Income Support, income-based Jobseekers Allowance or Family Credit (see page 129), you may be able to get a Maternity Payment to help buy things for your new baby. You can claim a Maternity Payment after the 29th week of pregnancy, up until the time your baby is three months old. If you're adopting a baby you can apply for Maternity Payment within three months of adoption, as long as the baby is not more than 12 months old when the application is made. Any savings over £500 will affect the amount of Maternity Payment you receive. Get claim form SF100 from an antenatal clinic or social security office.
- If you have a child under five years old and you're getting Income Support, or income-based Jobseeker's Allowance you'll automatically get a Cold Weather Payment for any consecutive seven-day period when the temperature averages 0°C or below. If you don't receive your payment, submit a written claim and ask for a decision.
- If you're getting Income Support or income-based Jobseeker's Allowance, you may be able to get a Community Care Grant. These non-repayable payments are given to help, for example, people with disabilities lead independent lives in the community. Sometimes grants are given to

families under exceptional stress. Grants may be made for items such as furniture and house repairs. Any savings of over £500 will affect the amount of Community Care Grant. Get form SF300 from your social security office.

- If you've been getting Income Support or income-based Jobseeker's Allowance for 26 weeks or more, you may be able to get a Budgeting Loan. These are interest-free loans made to help spread payment for certain expenses over a longer period. Loans may be made for items such as essential household equipment, safety equipment (such as a fireguard), furniture (such as bedding), repairs, and maintenance. The amount of the loan is decided by the Social Fund officer, according to your needs. The loan has to be repaid. Any savings over £500 will affect the amount of a Budgeting Loan. Get form SF300 from your social security office.

- In an emergency, if you can't afford something that's urgently needed, you may be able to get a Crisis Loan. These loans can cover living expenses for up to 14 days, or such things as essential household equipment or travel costs. Crisis Loans are only given if there's no other way of avoiding risk to somebody's health or safety. The amount of the loan is decided by the Social Fund officer. The loan has to be repaid.

For more information, contact a social security office.

FOR CHILDREN WITH SPECIAL NEEDS

If you've a disabled child who's needed a lot of extra looking after for at least three months, you may be able to get Disability Living Allowance. You can claim on form DLA1 Disability Living Allowance which you can get from your social security office or by ringing the number below.

If your child has difficulty walking or needs supervision and guidance outside, you can claim the mobility component of Disability Living Allowance from his or her fifth birthday.

If your child gets either the middle or the higher rate of the care component of Disability Living Allowance, and you spend a lot of time looking after him or her, you may also be able to get Invalid Care Allowance. You must be giving care for at least 35 hours a week and be earning less than a certain amount. DS700 Invalid Care Allowance claim pack tells you how to claim. You can get this from your social security office or by ringing the number below.

Your income-based Jobseeker's Allowance or Income Support will be increased if you get Disability Living Allowance for a dependent child.
There is a Benefit Enquiry Line for people with disabilities: Freephone 0800 882200 (in Northern Ireland, 0800 220674).

THE FAMILY FUND

The Family Fund is a government fund run by the Joseph Rowntree Foundation. It gives cash grants to families caring for children under 16 who have a severe physical or learning disability. Grants are made to meet special needs not met by the health or social services, for example, a washing machine, special equipment, clothing, bedding, holiday expenses. Family income and circumstances are taken into account when applications are considered, but there's no means test. Write to the address on page 136 for more information and an application form.

NEW DEAL FOR LONE PARENTS

What is it?
A new scheme for lone parents on income support with school age children offering advice and help in returning to work. NB The scheme is currently limited in availability but will become available nationally funded from October 1998.

How does it help?
With the provision of personal advisors to assist and support, lone parents can develop a personal plan of action for job search, training and childcare and identify the potential advantages of being in work rather than on benefits. Assistance will be given in building confidence, creating self esteem and gaining the relevant qualifications necessary for a return to work.

How to access the scheme
Contact your local job centre for advice about local availability of the scheme and for more information about getting back to work.

LEAFLETS
- *SB16 A guide to the Social Fund (in Northern Ireland, S16)*

USEFUL ORGANISATIONS

Some of these organisations are large; many are small. Some organisations have local branches; some can put you in touch with local groups.

Where there are separate addresses for Northern Ireland, Scotland and Wales, these are given. If an organisation doesn't cover the whole of the UK, the area is indicated: E, England; W, Wales; NI, Northern Ireland; S, Scotland.

Organisations marked * produce publications. When you write, it's usually a good idea to send a large stamped addressed envelope for a reply.

ADDICTIVE DRUGS

Drugaid (W)
64-66 Cardiff Road
Caerphilly CF83 1JQ
(01222) 881000
Provides counselling and information to drug/solvent misusers and the general public.

Narcotics Anonymous (UK service)
202 City Road
London EC1V 2PH
(0171) 251 4007
(0171) 730 0009
(Helpline 10am –10pm)
Self-help organisations whose members help each other to stay clear of drugs. Write or phone for information and the address of your local group. Some groups have a crèche.*

SCODA (The Standing Conference on Drug Abuse) (E, NI & W)
Waterbridge House
32-36 Loman Street
London SE1 0EE
(0171) 928 9500
In Scotland:
Scottish Drugs Forum
Shaftesbury House
5 Waterloo Street
Glasgow G2 6AY
(0141) 221 1175
Information on local treatment and services for drug users, family and friends.*

In England you can also ask the operator for Freefone Drug Problems which will give you a contact number for your local area. Or you can call the National Drugs Helpline on Freephone 0800 776600. In Wales you can also call Freephone 0800 371141 (Welsh). In Northern Ireland see Dunlewey Substance Advice Centre, Northlands and NICAS under Alcohol.

ALCOHOL

Alcohol Concern
Waterbridge House
32–36 Loman Street
London SE1 0EE
(0171) 928 7377
In Wales:
Welsh Drug and Alcohol Unit
4th Floor
St David's House
Wood Street
Cardiff CF1 1EY
(01222) 667766
For information on local alcohol councils offering advice, information, and support.*

Dunlewey Substance Advice Centre (NI)
226 Stewartstown Road
Belfast BT17 0LB
(01232) 611162
Help and personal counselling on alcohol, drug and solvent abuse.

Northern Ireland Community Addiction Service Ltd (NICAS) (NI)
40 Elmwood Avenue
Belfast BT9 6AZ
(01232) 664434
Counselling, treatment, education, information and training on dealing with alcohol and drug addiction.

Northlands (NI)
13 Pump Street
Londonderry BT48 6JG
(01504) 263356
For treatment, training, education and research about alcohol and other drug-related problems.

Scottish Council on Alcohol (S)
2nd Floor
166 Buchanan Street
Glasgow G1 2NH
(0141) 333 9677
For information about local councils on alcohol; promotes safer, healthier drinking styles; educates on alcohol-related problems.

BEHAVIOURAL DIFFICULTIES

SERENE (formerly CRY-SIS)
BM SERENE
London WC1N 3XX
(0171) 404 5011 (8am–11pm 7 days per week)
Self help and support for families with excessively crying, sleepless and demanding children.*

Enuresis Resource and Information Centre
34 Old School House
Britannia Road
Kingswood
Bristol BS15 8DB
(0117) 9603060 (9.30am–5.30pm Mon–Fri)
Provides advice and information to children, young adults, parents, and professionals on bed-wetting. Also sells bedding protection and enuresis alarms.

The Hyperactive Children's Support Group
Mrs S Bunday
71 Whyke Lane
Chichester PO19 2LD
(01903) 725182 (10am–1pm Monday–Friday)
Information to help problems related to hyperactivity and allergy.*

BREASTFEEDING

Association of Breastfeeding Mothers
PO Box 207
Bridgewater
Somerset TA6 7YT
(0181) 778 4769 (Recorded information)
Telephone advice service for breastfeeding mothers. Local support groups.*

La Leche League (Great Britain)
BM 3424
London WC1N 3XX
(0171) 242 1278
Help and information for women who want to breastfeed. Personal counselling. Local groups. Write with SAE for details of your nearest counsellor/group.*

National Childbirth Trust (NCT)
Alexandra House
Oldham Terrace
London W3 6NH
(0181) 992 8637
In Wales:
Contact (01222) 756239
Help, support and advice for mothers, including breastfeeding information and support, antenatal classes, postnatal groups. Write for details of your nearest branch.*

CHILDCARE/PLAY AND DEVELOPMENT

Child Growth Foundation
2 Mayfield Avenue, Chiswick
London W4 1PW
(0181) 994 7625
Information and advice for parents concerned about their child's growth.*

Mudiad Ysgolion Meithrin/ The National Association of Welsh Medium Nursery Schools and Playgroups (W)
145 Albany Road
Cardiff CF2 3NT
(01222) 485510
Help and advice on setting up and running parent and toddler groups and playgroups. Contact with local playgroups.

National Association for Maternal and Child Welfare (NAMCW)
40/42 Osnaburgh Street
London NW1 3ND
(0171) 383 4117
(0171) 383 4541
Advice and courses on child care and family life.*

National Association of Toy and Leisure
68 Churchway
London NW1 1LT
(0171) 387 9592
Information about local toy libraries (which lend toys). For all families with babies and young children, including those with special needs. Runs ACTIVE groups, which provide aids, information and workshops for children with disabilities.

Daycare Trust
Wesley House
4 Wild Court
London WC2B 4AU
(0171) 405 5617/8 (Helpline 9.30am–5.30pm Mon–Fri)
Campaigns for the provision of good childcare facilities. The Daycare Trust gives information on all aspects of childcare.*

National Childminding Association
8 Masons Hill
Bromley BR2 9EY
(0181) 464 6164
In Northern Ireland:
17A Court Street
Newtownards
Belfast BT23 3NX
(01247) 811015

In Scotland:
Scottish Childminding Association
National Development Officer
Room 7
Stirling Business Centre
Wellgreen
Stirling FK8 2DZ
(01786) 445377
An organisation for childminders, childcare workers, parents, and anyone with an interest in pre-school care. Works to improve status and conditions of childminders and standards of childcare.*

Parents at Work
45 Beech Street
London EC2Y 8AD
(0171) 628 3565
(Helpline 0171 628 3578)
Information and advice on childcare provision for working parents. Local groups.*

Pre-school Learning Alliance
69 King's Cross Road
London WC1X 9LL
(0171) 833 0991
In Northern Ireland:
NIPPA - The Early Years Organisation
Enterprise House
Boucher Crescent
Belfast BT12 6HU
(01232) 662825
In Scotland:
14 Elliot Place
Glasgow G3 8EP
(0141) 221 4148
In Wales:
2A Chester Street
Wrexham
Clwyd LL13 8BD
(01978) 358195
Help and advice on setting up and running parent and toddler groups and playgroups. Contact with local playgroups.

Working for Childcare (E, W & NI)
77 Holloway Road
London N7 8JZ
(0171) 700 0281
Advice and information for employers, trade unions, and others on workplace childcare.

CONTRACEPTION

Brook Advisory Centres (E, S & NI)
165 Gray's Inn Road
London WC1X 8UD
(0171) 713 9000
In Northern Ireland:
29a North Street
Belfast BT1 1NA
(01232) 328866
Advice and practical help with contraception and pregnancy testing, advice on unplanned pregnancies and sexual counselling for young men and women. Free and confidential. For your nearest centre look in the local phone book or contact Brook Central Office.*

Family Planning Association
2-12 Pentonville Road
London N1 9FP
(0171) 837 5432
In Northern Ireland:
113 University Street
Belfast BT7 1HP
(01232) 325488
In Wales:
4 Museum Place
Cardiff CF1 3BG
(01222) 342766
Information on all aspects of family planning and methods of contraception.*

Marie Stopes Clinic (E)
Marie Stopes House
108 Whitfield Street
London W1P 6BE
(0171) 388 0662
Registered charity providing family planning, women's health check-ups, male and female sterilisation, pregnancy testing, advice on unplanned pregnancies and sexual counselling for men and women. You don't need to be referred by your doctor, but you do need to book an appointment. A charge is made to cover costs. For centres in Manchester and Leeds look in the local phone book.*

DEPRESSION AND STRESS

Association for Postnatal Illness (APNI)
25 Jerdan Place
London SW6 1BE
(0171) 386 0868
(10am–5pm Mon–Fri)
Support for mothers suffering from postnatal depression.*

MAMA (Meet-a-mum Association)
26 Avenue Road
South Norwood
London SE25 4DX
(0181) 771 5595
In Wales:
Room 1
Mansel House
99 Mansel Street
Swansea SA1 5UE
Support for mothers suffering from postnatal depression or who feel lonely and isolated looking after a child at home. Will try to put you in touch with another mother who has experienced similar problems, or with a group of mothers locally, or help you to find ways of meeting people. Write with SAE for details of local groups.*

MIND (National Association for Mental Health)
Granta House
15–19 Broadway
London E15 4BQ
(0181) 522 1728
In Northern Ireland:
NI Association for Mental Health
Beacon House
80 University Street
Belfast BT7 1HE
(01232) 328474
In Wales:
23 St Mary Street
Cardiff CF1 2AA
(01222) 395123
Help for people with mental illness. Also advice and information about coming off anti-depressants, tranquillisers, etc. Local associations.

Parentline
Endway House
The Endway
Hadleigh,
Essex SS7 2AN
(01702) 554782
(01702) 559900 (Helpline 9am–9pm Mon–Fri, 1–6pm Sat)
Minicom 0800 783 6783
Support for troubled parents in times of stress or crisis, chiefly through a confidential and anonymous telephone helpline.

Parents Advice Centre (NI)
Franklin House
12 Brunswick Street
Belfast BT2 7GE
(01232) 238800
A confidential service offering support and guidance to parents under stress.

Scottish Association for Mental Health (S)
Atlantic House
38 Gardner's Crescent
Edinburgh EH3 8DQ
(0131) 229 9687
Network of local associations throughout Scotland.

HOUSING

Northern Ireland Housing Executive (NI)
2 Adelaide Street
Belfast BT2 8PB
(01232) 240588
Advice and information on all aspects of housing.

Shelter
88 Old Street
London EC1V 9HU
(0171) 253 0202
In Northern Ireland:
1-5 Coyles Place
Belfast BT7 1EL
(01232) 247752
In Scotland:
4th Floor
Scotia Bank House
6 South Charlotte Street
Edinburgh EH2 4AW
(0131) 473 7170
In Wales:
25 Walter Road
Swansea SA1 5NN
(01792) 469400
Help for those who are homeless and advice on any kind of housing problem.*

ILLNESS AND DISABILITY (GENERAL)

Action for Sick Children (NAWCH) (E & NI)
Argyle House
29-31 Euston Road
London NW1 2SD
(0171) 833 2041
In Scotland:
15 Smith's Place
Edinburgh EH6 8HT
(0131) 553 6553
In Wales:
The Association for the Welfare of Children in Hospitals (AWCH Wales)
4 Chestnut Avenue
West Cross
Swansea SA3 5NL
(01792) 404232
Support for sick children and their families – helping parents to be with their child in hospital and informing families about hospital care.*

Contact a Family
170 Tottenham Court Road
London W1P 0HA
(0171) 383 3555
Links families of children with special needs through contact lines. All disabilities. Local parent support groups.*

Disability Action (NI)
2 Annadale Avenue
Belfast BT7 3JH
(01232) 491011
Information and advice on physical disability and local organisations.

Disabled Living Foundation (DLF)
380-384 Harrow Road
London W9 2HU
(0171) 289 6111
In Northern Ireland:
Disabled Living Centre
Regional Disablement Services
Musgrave Park Hospital
Stockman's Lane
Belfast BT9 7JB
(01232) 669501 x2708

In Scotland:
Disability Scotland
Princes House
5 Shandwick Place
Edinburgh EH2 4RG
(0131) 229 8632
Information and advice on all aspects of disability, especially equipment and daily living problems. Referral to other organisations for adults and children with disabilities.*

MENCAP (Royal Society for Mentally Handicapped Children and Adults)
Mencap National Centre
123 Golden Lane
London EC1Y 0RT
(0171) 454 0454
In Northern Ireland:
Segal House
4 Annadale Avenue
Belfast BT7 3JH
(01232) 691351
In Wales:
31 Lambourne Crescent
Cardiff Business Park
Llanishen
Cardiff CF4 5GG
(01222) 747588
Information, support, and advice for parents of children with learning disabilities. Local branches.*

National Disability Advice
Line 0800 882200

Parentability
c/o National Childbirth Trust
A network within NCT specifically for the support of disabled parents

Royal Association for Disability and Rehabilitation (RADAR) (E)
12 City Forum
250 City Road
London EC1V 8AF
(0171) 250 3222
Information and advice on physical disability. Local organisations.*

ILLNESS AND DISABILITY (SPECIALISED)

Advisory Centre for Education (ACE) Ltd
Unit 1B
Aberdeen Studios
22-24 Highbury Grove
London N5 2DQ
(0171) 354 8318
(Business Line)
(0171) 354 8321
(Free advice line 2pm-5pm Mon-Fri)
Independent education advice service for parents and children with special needs.*

AFASIC – Association for All Speech Impaired Children
347 Central Markets
Smithfield
London EC1A 9NH
(0171) 236 3632/6487
In Northern Ireland:
28 Caulside Park
Newpark
Antrim BT41 2DS
(01849) 464849
In Wales:
6 Woodholm Close
Crundale
Haverfordwest
Pembroke SA62 4DH
(01437) 768771
Helps children with speech and language disorders. Information and advice for parents.*

Association for Spina Bifida and Hydrocephalus (ASBAH)
ASBAH House
42 Park Road
Peterborough PE1 2UQ
(01733) 555988

In Northern Ireland:
Graham House
Knockbraken Healthcare Park
Saintfield Road
Belfast BT8 8BH
(01232) 798878
In Wales:
(North Wales)
Canolfan yr Orsedd
Ffordd yr Orsedd
Llandudno
Gwynedd LL30 1LA
(01492) 878041
(South Wales)
4 Lakeside, Barry
South Glamorgan CF62 6SS
(01446) 735714
Support for parents of children with spina bifida and/or hydrocephalus. Advice, practical and financial help. Local groups.*

Association of Parents of Vaccine Damaged Children
78 Campden Lane
Shipston-on-Stour
Warwicks CV36 4DH
(01608) 661595
In Scotland:
21 Saughton Mains Gardens
Edinburgh EH11 3QG
(0131) 443 9287
Advises parents on claiming vaccine damage payment.

Body Positive
51B Philbeach Gardens
London SW5 9EB
(0171) 835 1045
(0171) 373 9124 (Helpline 7pm-10pm)
In Northern Ireland:
Room 308
Bryson House
28 Bedford Street
Belfast BT2 7FE
(01232) 235515 (2pm-4pm Tues-Fri)
In Scotland:
37-39 Montrose Terrace
Edinburgh EH7 5DJ
(0131) 652 0754
In Wales:
PO Box 237
Cardiff CF1 1XE
(01222) 343030
(Helpline Mon-Fri 10am-6.30pm)
Offers counselling and support services to those affected by HIV and AIDS, their families, partners and friends.

British Diabetic Association
10 Queen Anne Street
London W1M 0BD
(0171) 323 1531
In Northern Ireland:
John Gibson House
257 Lisburn Road
Belfast BT9 7EN
(01232) 666646
Information and support for all diabetics.*

Changing Faces
1-2 Junction Mews
London W2 1PN
(0171) 706 4232
Offers advice, information and support to carers of young children with facial disfigurements. Child specialist available to help young children cope.

Cleft Lip and Palate Association (CLAPA)
138 Buckingham Palace Road
London SW1W 9SA
(0121) 824 8110
Voluntary organisation of parents and professionals offering support to families of babies born with cleft lip and/or palate. Feeding equipment available. Local groups.*

Coeliac Society of the United Kingdom
PO Box 220
High Wycombe
Bucks HP11 2HY
(01494) 437278 (9.30am-3pm)
Helps parents of children diagnosed as having the coeliac condition or dermatitis herpetiformis.

Council for Disabled Children
8 Wakley Street
London EC1V 7QE
(0171) 843 6061
Information for parents and details of all organisations offering help with particular disabilities.

Cystic Fibrosis Trust
11 London Road
Bromley BR1 1BY
(0181) 464 7211
In Wales:
Cystic Fibrosis Trust Wales
WCVA
Llys Ifor
Crescent Road
Caerphilly CF8 1XL
(01222) 852751
Information and support for parents of children with cystic fibrosis and for people worried about the possibility of passing on the illness. Local groups.*

Down's Syndrome Association (E & W)
155 Mitcham Road
London SW17 9PG
(0181) 682 4001
In Scotland:
Scottish Down's Syndrome Association
158-160 Balgreen Road
Edinburgh EH11 3AU
(0131) 313 4225
In Northern Ireland:
Graham House
Knockbracken Healthcare Park
Saintfield Road
Belfast BT8 8BH
(01232) 704606
In Wales:
206 Whitchurch Road
Cardiff CF4 3NB
(01222) 522511
Information, advice, counselling and support for parents of children with Down's syndrome. Local groups. 24-hour helpline.*

Enable (Scottish Society for the Mentally Handicapped)
6th Floor
7 Buchanan Street
Glasgow G1 3HL
(0141) 226 4541
A comprehensive information and support service for people with learning difficulties.

Haemophilia Society
Chesterfield House
385 Euston Road
London NW1 3AU
(0171) 380 0600
In Northern Ireland:
Society House
6 Kilcoole Park
Belfast BT14 8LB
(01232) 729559
Information, advice and practical help for families affected by haemophilia. Some local groups.*

(I CAN) Invalid Children's Aid Nationwide (E & W)
Barbican City Gate
1-3 Dufferin Street
London EC1 8NA
(0171) 374 4422
Advice and information for parents of disabled children, especially those with severe speech and language disorders.

Meningitis Research Foundation
13 High Street
Thornbury
Bristol BS12 2AE
(01454) 413344

In Northern Ireland:
71a Botanic Avenue
Belfast BT7 1JL
(01232) 321283
In Scotland:
133 Gilmore Place
Edinburgh EH3 9PP
(0131) 228 3324
(01454) 413344 (24-hour national helpline)
Offers counselling for parents whose children have died from meningitis and gives support to people with loved ones in hospital or at home.*

Muscular Dystrophy Group
7-11 Prescott Place
London SW4 6BS
(0171) 720 8055
Support and advice through local branches and a network of Family Care Officers.

National AIDS Helpline
0800 567123
Calls are confidential, free and available 24 hours a day. There is a Minicom on 0800 521361 for people who are deaf or hard of hearing. Information in other languages:
Arabic - 0800 282447
(6 pm to 10 pm on Thursday);
Bengali - 0800 371132
(6 pm to 10 pm on Tuesday);
Cantonese - 0800 282446
(6 pm to 10 pm on Monday);
Gujarati - 0800 371134
(6 pm to 10 pm on Wednesday);
Hindi - 0800 371136
(6 pm to 10 pm on Wednesday);
Punjabi - 0800 371133
(6 pm to 10 pm on Wednesday);
Urdu - 0800 371135
(6 pm to 10 pm on Wednesday);
Welsh - 0800 371131
(10 am to 2 am daily). Leaflets can be ordered in all these languages.*
In Northern Ireland:
AIDS Helpline NI
0800 137437
7pm-10pm Mon-Fri and 2pm-5pm Sat

National Asthma Campaign
Providence House
Providence Place
London N1 0NT
(0171) 226 2260
0345 010203 Asthma helpline (9am-9pm each day)
In Northern Ireland:
124 Newry Road
Kilkeel BT34 4ET
(01693) 762811
Information and support for people with asthma, their families and health professionals. Booklets, videos and helpline. Over 180 nationwide branches.*

National Autistic Society
393 City Road
London EC1V 1NE
(0171) 833 2299
(0171) 903 3555 (Advice line 10am-12pm Mon-Fri)
In Northern Ireland:
Parents and Professionals in Autism (PAPA) (NI)
Graham House
Knockbraken Healthcare Park
Saintfield Road
Belfast BT8 8BH
(01232) 401729
Provides day and residential centres for the care and education of autistic children. Puts parents in touch with one another. Information and advice.

National Deaf Children's Society (NDCS)
15 Dufferin Street
London EC1Y 8PD
(0171) 490 8656
(0171) 250 0123
(Helpline 10am–5pm Mon–Fri,
Tues 10am–7pm)
In Northern Ireland:
Wilton House
5 College Square North
Belfast BT1 6AR
(01232) 313170 (voice and text)
Works for deaf children and their
families. Information and advice on all
aspects of childhood deafness. Local
self-help groups.*

National Eczema Society (NES)
163 Eversholt Street
London NW1 1BU
(0171) 388 4097
In Northern Ireland:
9 Nottinghill
Malone Road
Belfast BT9 5NS
(01232) 666393 (after 6pm)
Support and information for people
with eczema and their families.
Nationwide network of local contacts
offering practical advice and support.*

National Meningitis Trust
Fern House, Bath Road
Stroud GL5 3TJ
(01453) 751738
0345 538118 (24 hour helpline)
In Wales
149 The Hawthorns
Brackla
Bridgend CF31 2PG
(01656) 656713
Information and support for those
already affected by meningitis. Local
groups.

**Northern Ireland Council for
Orthopaedic Development
(NICOD) (NI)**
Malcolm Sinclair House
31 Ulsterville Avenue
Belfast BT9 7AS
(01232) 666188
Advice and support for parents of
children with cerebral palsy.*

Positively Women (E)
347-349 City Road
London EC1V 1LR
(0171) 713 0222 (Helpline Mon-
Fri 10am–4pm)
(0171) 713 0444 (Admin)
Offers counselling and support
services to women who are HIV
positive.*

**Reach (The Association for
Children with Hand or Arm
Deficiency)**
12 Wilson Way
Earls Barton
Northamptonshire NN6 0NZ
(01604) 811041
Information and support to parents of
children with hand or arm problems.
Can put you in touch with individual
families in a similar situation or local
groups.*

**Research Trust for Metabolic
Diseases in Children (RTMDC)**
Golden Gates Lodge
Weston Road
Crewe CW2 5XN
(01270) 250221 (office hours
answerphone after hours for
urgent calls)
Makes grants and allowances for the
medical treatment and care of
children with metabolic diseases. Puts
parents in touch with each other.

Restricted Growth Association
PO Box 8
Countesthorpe
Leicester LE8 5ZS
(0116) 247 8913
Offers support to parents who have a
child with growth problems.*

**Royal National Institute for the
Blind (RNIB)**
224 Great Portland Street
London W1N 6AA
(0171) 388 1266
In Northern Ireland:
40 Linenhall Street
Belfast BT2 8BG
(01232) 329373
In Scotland:
9 Viewfield Place
Stirling FK8 1NL
(01786) 451752 (Resource
Centre)
In Wales:
14 Neville Street, Canton
Cardiff CF1 8UX
(01222) 224574
Information, advice and services for
blind people.

**Royal National Institute for the
Deaf (RNID)**
19-20 Featherstone Street
London EC1Y 8SL
(0171) 296 8000
(0171) 296 8001 minicom
In Northern Ireland:
Wilton House
5 College Square North
Belfast BT1 6AR
(01232) 239619 (voice and text)
In Wales:
3rd Floor
33-35 Cathedral Road
Cardiff CF1 9HB
(01222) 333034
Minicom (01222) 333036
Information, advice and services for
deaf and hard of hearing people.

SCOPE
6 Market Road
London N7 9PW
(0171) 636 5020
(0800) 626216 (E and W helpline
Mon-Fri 9 am–9 pm;
2 pm–6 pm weekends)
In Wales:
Wales Regional Centre
Links Court Business Park
St Mellons
Cardiff
(01222) 797706
Offers advice and support to parents
of children with cerebral palsy.*
In Scotland
Capability Scotland
11 Ellersly Road
Edinburgh EH12 6HY
(0131) 313 5510

**Scottish Society for Autistic
Children (S)**
Hilton House
Alloa Business Park
Whins Road
Alloa FK10 3SA
(01259) 720044
Provides day and residential centres
for the care and education of autistic
children. Support groups. Information
and advice.*

**SENSE (National Deaf-Blind and
Rubella Association)**
11–13 Clifton Terrace
Finsbury Park
London N4 3SR
(0171) 272 7774
In Northern Ireland:
The Manor House
51 Mallusk Road
Mallusk BT37 9AA
(01232) 833430

In Scotland:
Head Office
Unit 5/2
8 Elliot Place
Clydeway Centre
Glasgow G3 8EP
(0141) 221 7577 (voice)
Advice and support for families of
deaf-blind and rubella-disabled
children.*

Sickle Cell Society
54 Station Road
Harlesden
London NW10 4UA
(0181) 961 7795/4006
Information, advice and counselling
for families affected by sickle cell
disease or trait. Financial help when
needed.

**Sickle Cell and Thalassaemia
Centre (W)**
Bute Town Health Centre
Loudoun Square
Butetown
Cardiff CF1 5UZ
(01222) 471055
Information, advice, and counselling
for families affected by sickle cell
disease or trait. Financial help when
needed.*

The Toxoplasmosis Trust
61–71 Collier Street
London N1 9BE
(0171) 713 0599 (Helpline)
Information and advice for pregnant
women and support and counselling
for sufferers and their families.

The UK Thalassaemia Society
19 The Broadway
Southgate Circus
London N14 6PH
(0181) 882 0011
Information, and advice for families
affected by thalassaemia.*

Wales Council for the Blind (W)
Shand House
20 Newport Road
Cardiff CF2 1DB
(01222) 473954
Information, advice and services for
blind people.

LONE PARENTS

Gingerbread
16–17 Clerkenwell Close
London EC1R 0AA
(0171) 336 8183
In Northern Ireland:
169 University Street
Belfast BT7 1HR
(01232) 231417
In Scotland:
304 Maryhill Road
Glasgow G20 7YE
(0141) 353 0989
In Wales:
Room 1, Mansel House
99 Mansel Street
Swansea SA1 5UE
(01792) 648728
(9am-3.30pm Tuesday and
Wednesday, 9am - 12pm Friday).
Self-help association for one-parent
families. Local groups offer support,
friendship, information, advice and
practical help.

LOSS AND
BEREAVEMENT

Compassionate Friends
53 North Street
Bristol BS3 1EN
(0117) 953 9639
An organisation of and for bereaved
parents. Advice and support. Local
groups.*

CRUSE (E & S)
126 Sheen Road
Richmond
Surrey TW9 1UR
(0181) 332 7227 (Helpline)
(0181) 940 4818 (Office)
In Northern Ireland:
Piney Ridge
Knockbracken Healthcare Park
Saintfield Road
Belfast BT8 8BH
(01232) 792419
In Wales:
Old Bedw
Builth Wells
Powys LD2 3LQ
(01982) 560468
Offers help and counselling to
bereaved people. Local groups.

**Foundation for the Study of
Infant Deaths (Cot Death
Research and Support)**
14 Halkin Street
London SW1X 7DP
(0171) 235 0965 (Helpline)
In Northern Ireland:
Friends of the Foundation for the
Study of Infant Deaths (Northern
Ireland)
7 Glenann Avenue
Belfast BT17 9AT
(01232) 622688
Support and information for parents
bereaved by a sudden infant death.*

Scottish Cot Death Trust (S)
Royal Hospital for Sick Children
Yorkhill
Glasgow G3 8SJ
(0141) 357 3946
Support and information for parents
bereaved by sudden infant death. Puts
parents in touch with local support
groups of other bereaved parents.*

**Stillbirth and Neonatal Death
Society (SANDS)**
28 Portland Place
London W1N 4DE
(0171) 436 5881 (9.30am–5.00pm
Mon–Fri) Information and a national
network of support groups for
bereaved parents. Phone or write for
details.*

RELATIONSHIPS

**RELATE: National Marriage
Guidance**
Herbert Gray College
Little Church Street
Rugby CV21 3AP
(01788) 573241
In Northern Ireland:
76 Dublin Road
Belfast BT2 7HP
(01232) 323454
Confidential counselling on
relationship problems of any kind. To
find your local branch look under
RELATE or Marriage Guidance in the
phone book or contact the above
addresses.

RIGHTS AND
BENEFITS/ACCESS TO
SERVICES

Child Poverty Action Group
4th Floor
1–5 Bath Street
London EC1V 9PY
(0171) 253 3406
In Northern Ireland:
12 Queen Street
Londonderry BT48 7EG
(01504) 267777
Campaigns on behalf of low-income
families. Provides advisers with
information and advice for parents on
benefits, housing, welfare rights, etc.*

Child Support Agency
PO Box 55
Brierley Hill
West Midlands DY5 1YL
0345 133133 (enquiry line)
In Northern Ireland:
Great Northern Tower
Great Victoria Street
Belfast BT2 7AD
0345 132615
The Government agency that assesses
maintenance levels for parents who
no longer live with their children. The
agency will claim maintenance on
behalf of the parent with care of the
children but if you are on benefits the
money claimed will be deducted from
your benefit.

Citizen's Advice Bureaux
National Association of Citizen's
Advice Bureaux
Myddleton House
115–123 Pentonville Road
London N1 9LZ
(0171) 833 2181
In Northern Ireland:
11 Upper Crescent
Belfast BT7 1NT
(01232) 739447
In Scotland:
26 George Square
Edinburgh EH8 9LD
(0131) 667 0156
In North Wales:
Unit 7, St Asaph Business Park
Glascoed
St Asaph
Denbighshire LL17 0LJ
In South Wales:
Ground Floor, Quebec House
Castlebridge
5-19 Cowbridge Road East
Cardiff CF1 9AB
For advice on all benefits, housing,
your rights generally, and many other
problems. To find your local CAB
look in the phone book, ask at your
local library, or contact one of the
head offices for the address. There
may also be other advice centres in
your area offering similar help.

Community Health Councils
CHCs exist to help users of NHS.
They advise on where and how to get
the service you need, and can help if
you've a complaint.
In Scotland CHCs are called Local
Health Councils; in Northern Ireland,
Health and Social Services Councils.
For your local CHC, look in your
phone book under the name of your
district health authority/ health
board/local Health and Social Services
Council.

**Community Relations Councils
(CRCs)**
Commission for Racial Equality
10–12 Allington Street
London SW1E 5EH
(0171) 828 7022
In Northern Ireland:
Glendinning House
6 Murray Street
Belfast BT1 6DN
(01232) 439953
In Wales:
Community Relations for Racial
Equality
Unit 8
William Court
Trade Street
Cardiff CF1 5DQ
(01222) 224097
Sometimes called Councils for Racial
Equality or Community Relations
Offices. They are concerned with
community relations in their area and
often know of local minority ethnic
organisations and support groups. To
find your CRC look in your phone
book, ask at your town hall or local
library, or contact the above.

Disability Alliance Educational and Research Association
Universal House
88–94 Wentworth Street
London E1 7SA
(0171) 247 8763 (Advice line Mon, Wed 2pm–4pm, Tues, Thu, Fri 10am–4pm)
(0171) 247 8776
Information and advice on benefits for all people with disabilities. Publishes the *Disability Rights Handbook* – an annual guide to rights, benefits and services for those with disabilities and their families.

Family Fund
PO Box 50
York YO1 2ZX
(01904) 621115
A government fund independently administered by the Joseph Rowntree Memorial Trust. Gives cash grants to families caring for severely disabled children under 16.

Health Information Wales
Ffynnon-las
Ty Glas Avenue
Llanishen
Cardiff CF4 5DZ
0800 665544 (Freephone 9am–5pm with Minicom)
A confidential information service on health matters. Provides details of self-help groups in your area.

Maternity Alliance
45 Beech Street
London EC2P 2LX
(0171) 588 8582 (10am–1pm Mon–Thu)
Information on all aspects of maternity care and rights. Advice on benefits, maternity rights at work.*

National Council for One Parent Families
255 Kentish Town Road
London NW5 2LX
(0171) 267 1361
Free information for one-parent families on financial, legal and housing problems.*

NHS Helpline (S)
Network Scotland
57 Ruthven Lane
Glasgow G12 9JQ
0800 224488
Provides information about health services and the NHS in Scotland. Calls are free and confidential. Free leaflets also available on a wide range of health topics.

Social Security: Freeline
For general advice on all social security benefits, pensions and National Insurance including maternity benefits and Income Support, phone Freeline Social Security on 0800 666555 between 9am and 4.30pm on weekdays, and between 9am and 1pm Saturdays. Calls are free. There is an answerphone service out of hours.
Advice in Urdu or Punjabi:
Phone Freeline 0800 289188 between 9am and 4pm weekdays.
For *Punjabi* only telephone Freeline 0800 521360 during the same hours.

Social security: local offices
For general advice on all social security benefits, pensions and National Insurance, including maternity benefits and Income Support and Income-based Jobseeker's Allowance, telephone, write or call in to your local social security office. The address will be in the phone book under 'social security'. Hours are usually 9.30am to 3.30pm. In busy offices there may be a very long wait if you call in.

Social services
A social worker at your local social services office will give you information on topics including benefits, housing, financial difficulties, employment, relationship problems, childcare and useful organisations. Look up social services in the phone book under the name of your local authority or ask at your local library. Phone, write or call in. There may also be a social worker based at the hospital to whom you could talk either during your antenatal care or when you or your baby are in hospital. Ask your midwife or other hospital staff to put you in contact.

SAFETY AND FIRST AID

British Red Cross Society (BRCS)
9 Grosvenor Crescent
London SW1X 7EJ
(0171) 235 5454
In Northern Ireland:
87 University Street
Belfast BT7 1HP
(01232) 246400
In Scotland:
Alexandra House
204 Bath Street
Glasgow G2 4HL
(0141) 332 9591
In Wales:
Llys Ifor
Crescent Road
Caerphilly
Mid Glamorgan CF8 1LX
(01222) 810021
Among other activities, runs first aid courses through local branches. Look under British Red Cross or Red Cross in the phone book or contact the above address.*

Child Accident Prevention Trust (CAPT)
18–20 Farringdon Lane
London EC1R 3AU
(0171) 608 3828
In Northern Ireland:
Department of Epidemiology
Mulhouse Building
Grosvenor Road
Belfast BT12 6BJ
(01232) 240503 x2588
Promotes child safety. Help and advice for parents.*

NSPCC (National Society for the Prevention of Cruelty to Children)
42 Curtain Road
London EC2A 3NH
(0171) 825 2500
0800 800500 (free national helpline)
In Northern Ireland:
Jennymount Court
North Derby Street
Belfast BT15 3HN
(01232) 351135
Aims to prevent all forms of child abuse. If you're in need of help or know of anyone who needs help, look in the phone book for the number of your nearest NSPCC office.*

Parents Anonymous
6–9 Manor Gardens
London N7 6LA
(0171) 263 8918
A 24-hour telephone answering service Monday to Friday for parents who feel they can't cope or who feel they might abuse their children.

The Royal Life Saving Society UK
River House
High Street
Broom
Warwickshire B50 4HN
(01789) 773994
e-mail: mail@rlss.org.uk
Runs courses on baby resuscitation. Send sae for leaflet *Save a baby's life.*

The Royal Society for the Prevention of Accidents (RoSPA)
Edgbaston Park
353 Bristol Road
Birmingham B5 7ST
(0121) 248 2000
In Northern Ireland:
117 Lisburn Road
Belfast BT9 7BS
(01232) 669453
In Scotland:
Slateford House
53 Lanarck Road
Edinburgh EH14 1TL
(0131) 455 7457
In Wales:
7 Cleeve House
Lambourne Crescent
Cardiff CF4 5GJ
(01222) 762529
Advice on the prevention of accidents of all kinds. Runs the Tufty Club for under five-year-olds.*

St John Ambulance
1 Grosvenor Crescent
London SW1X 7EF
(0171) 235 5231
In Northern Ireland:
Erne
Knockbracken Healthcare Park
Saintfield Road
Belfast BT8 8RA
(01232) 799393
In Scotland:
St Andrew's Ambulance Association
St Andrew's House
48 Milton Street
Glasgow G4 0HR
(0141) 332 4031
In Wales:
Priory House
Meridian Court
North Road
Cardiff CF4 3BL
(01222) 627627
Runs local first aid courses. Look for your nearest branch in the phone book, or contact the above address.*

SMOKING

ASH
16 Fitzhardinge Street
London W1H 9PL
(0171) 224 0743
In Scotland:
8 Frederick Street
Edinburgh EH2 2HB
(0131) 225 4725
In Wales:
372A Cowbridge Road East
Cardiff CF5 1HE
(01222) 641101
Assists smokers wishing to stop and promotes non-smoking as the norm in society. Information and resource centre for the public.*

Quitline
0800 00 22 00
Quitline in Wales
0345 697500
Advice on stopping smoking and details of local stop- smoking support services. Phone between 9.30am and 5.30pm on weekdays. Recorded advice available at other times. Or if you prefer to write for information:
Quit * (E)
Victory House
170 Tottenham Court Road
London W1P 0HA
(0171) 388 5775

Smokeline (S)
Network Scotland
Ruthven Lane
Glasgow G12 9JQ
0800 848484 (freephone 12pm–12am every day)
Provides support and encouragement to those who wish to stop smoking or who have recently stopped and want to stay stopped. Callers can receive a free *You can stop smoking* booklet.*

Ulster Cancer Foundation (NI)
40–42 Eglantine Avenue
Belfast BT9 6DX
(01232) 663281
Carries out cancer research and education programmes in Northern Ireland. Also provides information on the dangers of smoking and advice and support to smokers who want to quit.

SUPPORT AND INFORMATION

Equal Opportunities Commission
Overseas House
Quay Street
Manchester M3 3HN
(0161) 833 9244
In Northern Ireland:
Chamber of Commerce House
22 Great Victoria Street
Belfast BT2 7BA
(01232) 242752
Information and advice on issues of discrimination and equal opportunities.*

Family Welfare Association
501–505 Kingsland Road
London E8 4AU
(0171) 254 6251
National charity providing free social work services, e.g. counselling for relationship difficulties and advice on benefits, housing and other problems. Provides grants for people in need throughout the UK.*

Home-Start UK
2 Salisbury Road
Leicester LE1 7QR
(0116) 233 9955
In Northern Ireland:
133 Bloomfield Avenue
Belfast BT5 5AB
(01232) 460772
A voluntary home-visiting scheme. Volunteers visit families with children under five and offer friendship, practical help, and emotional support. Write for list of local schemes.

Institute for Complementary Medicine
PO Box 194
London SE16 1QZ
(0171) 237 5165
Charity providing information on complementary medicine and referrals to qualified practitioners or helpful organisations.*

The Multiple Births Foundation
Queen Charlotte's and Chelsea Hospital
Goldhawk Road
London W6 0XG
(0181) 383 3519
For professional support of families with twins and multiple births.

Parent Network (E)
Room 2
Winchester House
11 Cranmer Road
London SW9 6EJ
(0171) 735 1214 (10am–4pm Mon–Fri)
Runs Parent-link groups, which offer a listening ear and ideas on handling recurring daily situations that all parents face. Local support groups, newsletters and videos.

Patients' Association
PO Box 935
Harrow
Middlesex HA1 3YJ
(0181) 423 8999
Advice service for patients who have difficulties with their doctor. *

Twins and Multiple Births Association (TAMBA)
Harnott House
Little Sutton
South Wirral L66 1QQ
(0151) 348 0020 or
0870 121 4000
TAMBA Twinline (Helpline) (01732) 868000 (7 pm to 11 pm weekdays; 10 am to 10 pm weekends)
Advice and support for parents of multiples. Network of local Twins Clubs.*

Women's Aid Federation England
PO Box 391
Bristol BS99 7WS
(01179) 444411 (Adminstration Mon–Thu 10am–5pm, Fri 10am–3pm)
(0345) 023468 (helpline)
In Northern Ireland:
129 University Street
Belfast BT7 1HP
(01232) 249041
In Scotland:
12 Torphichen Street
Edinburgh EH3 8JQ
(0131) 221 0401 (10am–1pm)
In Wales:
4 Pound Place
Aberystwyth
Ceredigion SY23 1LX
(01970) 612748 (10am–4pm Mon–Fri)
or
38 –48 Crwys Road
Cardiff
South Glamorgan
CF2 4NN
(01222) 390874/390878
or
1st Floor
26 Wellington Road
Rhyl
Clwyd LL18 1BN
(01745) 334767
or
Glyndwr Women's Aid
12-14 Hall Square
Denbigh
Denbighshire
(01745) 814454
or
SNAP Cymru
45 Penarth Road
Cardiff CF1 5DJ
(01222) 388776 (9am–5pm)
Information, support and refuge for abused women and their children.

Women's Health
52 Featherstone Street
London EC1Y 8RT
(0171) 251 6580 (call 10am–4pm, not open Tuesday)
Information and support on many aspects of women's health. Provides a network of individual women who support others with similar health problems.*